Women'sHealth
FLAT BELLY
WORKOUTS

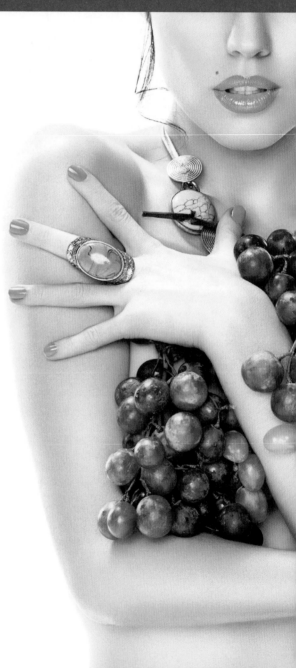

EDITOR-IN-CHIEF FARRAH STORR

EDITOR TOM STONE

ART DIRECTOR GRAEME SAPSED

SUB EDITORS BETH WILSON
LUCY TREVALLION
SCARLETT WRENCH

PRODUCTION ROGER BILSLAND

Top of every woman's body wish list is a flat belly. A taught, toned tummy ensures you ooze confidence whatever you're wearing: whether that's your weekend jeans, a party dress or a bikini. It's also the ultimate badge of health and vitality: once you've got a sexy stomach, your motivation to keep working out will skyrocket. It's a virtuous circle. But how do you get one in the first place? That's the question *Women's Health* readers ask most often. And that's why we decided to put together this comprehensive guide to achieving just that. Using the simple workout moves and nutrition rules in this book, anyone can sculpt the body of their dreams in just a few weeks. So what are you waiting for?

ENTS

A better body begins with loving the right foods

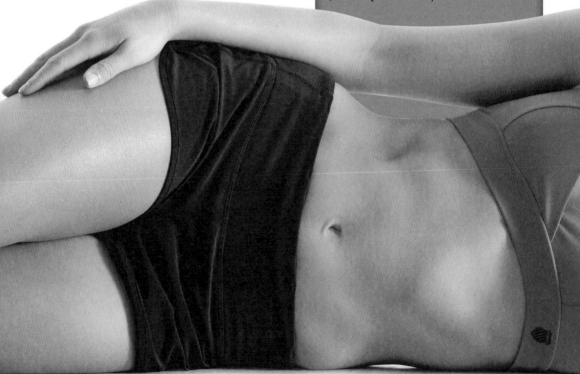

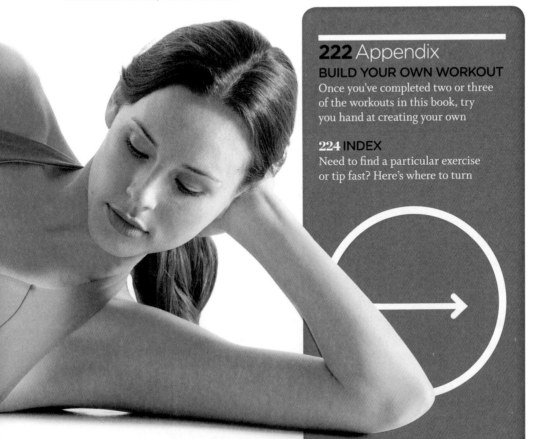

THE LATEST HOT-BODY NEWS

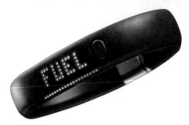

FIGHT FAT WITH TECHNOLOGY

Shame on us. A new study found women exercised for an average of just 18 minutes a day, while men did the recommended 30. Use the new Nike FuelBand bracelet (£129, nike.com) to track your activity levels, then chart your progress online. Fuel proof.

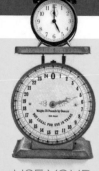

USE YOUR ALARM TO GET LIGHTER

A new study in the *American Journal of Health Promotion* found that women who wake up at a consistent time each day had lower body fat: those with more than 90 minutes of variation in their wake times had higher body fat than those with less than 60 minutes of variation. Professor Bailey, who led the study says, "Sleeping-in may be doing more harm than good." Bailey also found that the length of time you sleep affects your body fat levels. Forget 8-10 hours, it seems 8-8.5 hours is ideal, as longer in bed can also lead to more fat storage. Simply leave your weekday alarm set to the same time at the weekend to reap the rewards.

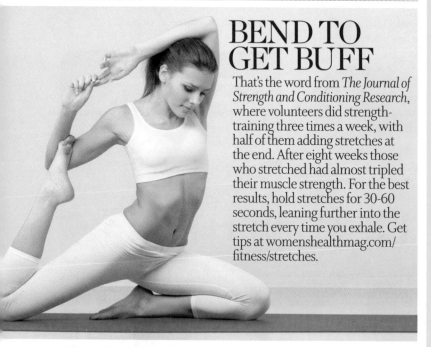

BEND TO GET BUFF

That's the word from *The Journal of Strength and Conditioning Research*, where volunteers did strength-training three times a week, with half of them adding stretches at the end. After eight weeks those who stretched had almost tripled their muscle strength. For the best results, hold stretches for 30-60 seconds, leaning further into the stretch every time you exhale. Get tips at womenshealthmag.com/fitness/stretches.

72

The percentage of each day that the average person's muscles are inactive – even if you're a gym bunny. Our advice: sneak in some stealth exercises such as bottom clenches on the bus or lifting your legs out under your desk. You can even firm up your jawline by doing facial exercises on the loo – get the moves at evafraser.com.

UNIVERSITY OF JYVASKYLA, FINLAND

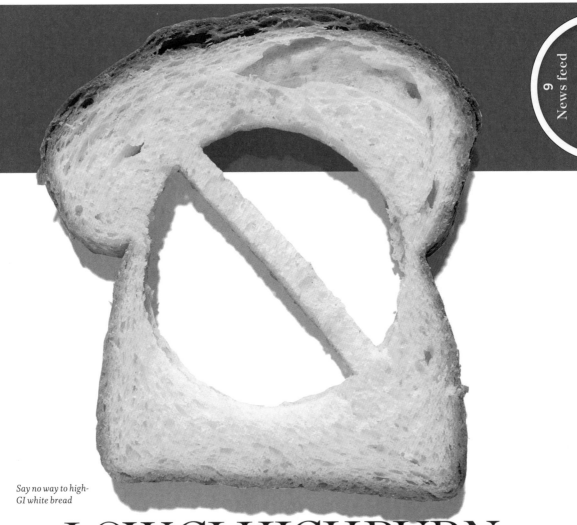

Say no way to high-GI white bread

LOW GI, HIGH BURN

Like metabolisms, not all calories are created equal. A Harvard Medical School study found low-glycemic diets – think lentils, whole grains and other foods that keep your blood sugar level – are more effective than low-fat or low-carb diets at burning calories. If we did a medal ceremony of GI foods, anything with a GI rating of 55 and below would get a gold, between 55 and 70 is silver, while over 70 doesn't even finish the race. Get GI ratings for any foods with the My Glycemic Index app (£2.49). Pure GI-nius.

GET OFF AND SHAPE UP

Exciting news: Indiana University found 40% of women have had an orgasm during a workout. While there's no magic formula, the best moves are core exercises and yoga. Try strengthening pelvic muscles with gluteal bridges: lie on your back, arms at your sides and knees bent. Raise your hips and hold. Core blimey.

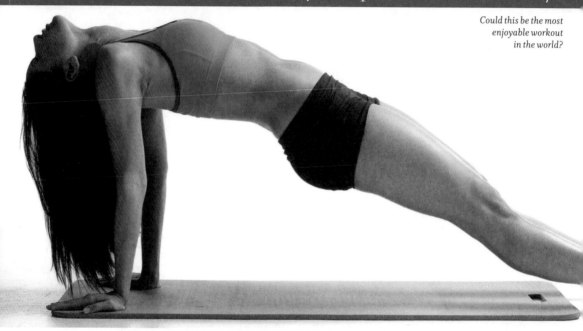

Could this be the most enjoyable workout in the world?

PUT A POSITIVE SPIN ON YOUR CYCLE

That time of the month shouldn't stop you exercising altogether, but it's a good idea to ease off pavement pounding the week before your period. Research shows nerve fibres around the knee fire more often then, affecting joint stability and upping your risk of injury. Ouch. It's not all bad though. Here's how you can alter your workout routine when Aunt Flo comes to town.

1 Do weights like a dude
During your period, your levels of oestrogen and progesterone drop, so your body is, ironically, more like a man's. Use that extra strength and hit the weights.

2 Swim your belly off
Research shows a 20-minute swim can deflate monthly bloat as the water pressure sends extra fluid back into your bloodstream. Breaststroke works best.

3 Flake out, tone up
Rest for a week mid-cycle, when your hormones peak. A study found you'll get better results if you chill, then lift weights every other day the rest of the time.

I'm milking it!

4 Milk your metabolic boost
You burn up to 359 more calories a day in the week before your period, according to a US study. Fuel up with dairy – calcium can cut PMS symptoms.

15

The number of pounds you gain in one year alone by drinking just one can of sugar-sweetened soft drink a day. That's more than a stone on fizzy pop alone. Got a sweet tooth? Try Zeo (£4.29 for 4, Ocado.com) for an all-natural fizz that has low levels of sugar extracted from sugar beets and stevia. And none of the artificial nasties you'll find in regular diet drinks. Cheers!

11 News feed

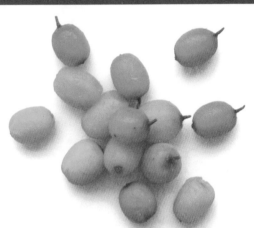

THE NEW SUPER FRUIT
SEA BUCKTHORN

This grape-sized orange berry is not only extremely tasty it also aids weight loss to boot. A Canadian study found it's packed with flab-busting omega-3 fatty acids, as well as health boosting antioxidant vitamins A, K, E and C. You can buy the dried version now from healthysupplies.co.uk (£4.99 for 100g). Get ready to buck up.

4

The hours of training you need each week to get better at a sport. Improve further with the Coach's Eye app (£2.99). Upload a clip of your performance and get advice from sports pros. Oh, did we mention the fat-burning benefits of all that practice?

BUILD CONFIDENCE, CARVE MUSCLES

A brave new world of exercise classes is hitting a gym near you. We asked the experts to explain what's involved and how they can improve your workout

2

The number of coffees it takes to cut post-workout muscle soreness by 48%. Caffeine blocks the brain's receptors for adrenose, the chemical that causes soreness. Try two cups an hour before working out.
SOURCE: JOURNAL OF PAIN

INDO ROW
SAY WHAT? "In this interval-based class, you work as part of a 'rowing crew' doing a series of drills of varying intensities," says former World Champion oarsman Josh Crosby.
BEST FOR Calorie burning – a 50-minute class blasts 800kcal.
BODY TARGET Shoulders and abs.
FIND IT waterrower.com/indorow

VIPR VIBE
SAY WHAT? The ViPR is that odd-looking rubber tube you'll have spotted being swung about at the gym. In the Vibe class, you use it on a Power Plate for extra exertion, says trainer Steve Powell.
BEST FOR Building muscles. Plus, you burn 400 calories a pop.
BODY TARGET Toning your legs and arms.
FIND IT powerplate.com/uk

GLOW YOGA
SAY WHAT? "It's a flow yoga class taught in an infrared heated studio," says instructor Nahid De Belgeonne. The heat is gentler than in Bikram yoga, so your body eases into the moves more easily.
BEST FOR Posture and beating stress, plus you'll use 400 calories.
BODY TARGET Leaner legs and a tighter core.
FIND IT goodvibesfitness.co.uk

2.75

THE NUMBER OF TIMES GREATER YOUR RISK OF HEART-RELATED DEATH IF YOU HAVE A NORMAL BMI BUT A FAT BELLY, COMPARED TO A NORMAL HIP-TO-WAIST RATIO (DIVIDE YOUR WAIST SIZE BY YOUR HIPS). ANYTHING OVER 0.8 IS RISKY – ACT NOW.

US NATIONAL CANCER INSTITUTE

PENCIL IN GYM VISITS TO GET AHEAD

Studying? Make sure you work out. Purdue University researchers compared the number of gym visits to exam results. "Students who sweated it out at least once a week were more likely to earn a higher average grade than those who visited less," says Tricia Zelaya from Purdue's Division of Recreational Sports. "They also had better time management skills." So it is possible to have brains and brawn.

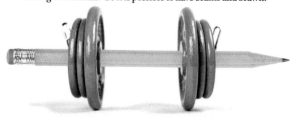

BIKER BRAIN

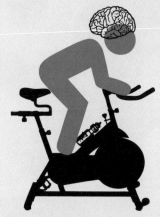

If you struggle to remember your Twitter password, get cycling. Researchers found just six minutes on a spin bike enhances memory, possibly thanks to the release of noradrenaline, a chemical messenger that contributes to brain storage. On yer bike!

UNIVERSITY OF CALIFORNIA, IRVINE

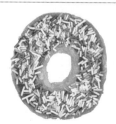

CUT CRAVINGS AT THE GYM

Tempted to blow your diet this weekend? Head to the gym and get a sweat on. Research has found the natural high induced by an hour of exercise will dampen your desire for a Sunday afternoon doughnut-fest (yes, we crave them, too) and reduce how much you eat. Added bonus: no more guilt come Monday. How sweet is that?

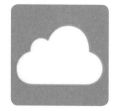

AVOID SKY-HIGH DIET HOPES

Slow and steady wins the weight-loss race. New research found lofty diet expectations can lead to yo-yo losses and a drop in confidence, says study author Dr Erin Olson. The Dream A Bit app (69p, iTunes) will help you stay on track. Start with small realistic goals, such as, "I will eat a vegetable at every meal." The tortoise would approve.

THREE

THE PERCENTAGE INCLINE ON THE TREADMILL THAT BEST SIMULATES OUTDOOR HIKING. FOR THE TRULY AMBITIOUS AMONG YOU, ADD 2LB ANKLE WEIGHTS TO YOUR WORKOUT TO FEEL LIKE YOU'RE HOT-FOOTING IT UP THE ALPS. LEDERHOSEN OPTIONAL.

THE JOURNAL OF STRENGTH & CONDITIONING RESEARCH

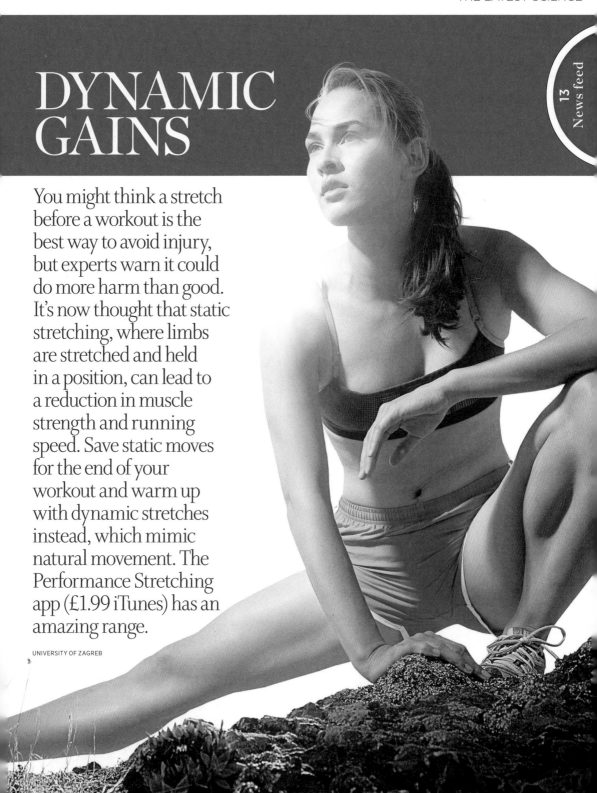

DYNAMIC GAINS

You might think a stretch before a workout is the best way to avoid injury, but experts warn it could do more harm than good. It's now thought that static stretching, where limbs are stretched and held in a position, can lead to a reduction in muscle strength and running speed. Save static moves for the end of your workout and warm up with dynamic stretches instead, which mimic natural movement. The Performance Stretching app (£1.99 iTunes) has an amazing range.

UNIVERSITY OF ZAGREB

WORK YOUR HEART WITH WEIGHTS

It sculpts your guns but heaving weights also gives your heart a workout. Researchers pitted kettlebell against treadmill workouts. Both an improved cardio fitness equally but strength training revved metabolisms for extra fat burning long after the workout was over. Which explains why the workouts in this book are super effective, without a treadmill in sight.

SOURCE: JOURNAL OF STRENGTH AND CONDITIONING RESEARCH

AVERAGE HEART RATE	Kettlebell **180** Treadmill **177**
AVERAGE RESPIRATORY RATE (breaths per minute)	Kettlebell **36** Treadmill **38**

BEAT THE MENU

Would a burger appeal if you knew you'd have to sprint for 33 minutes to burn it off? Studies at Texas Christian University show listing calories doesn't make people order lighter options, but listing the exercise needed does. Here's how your favourite foods stack up...

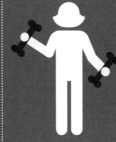

BONE UP BEFORE A WORKOUT

Timing is everything. Eating calcium before working out helps minimise exercise-induced calcium and bone-density loss through sweat. Eat a calcium-rich snack such as a yoghurt or nuts 30 minutes before training to protect your joints. Cracking.

15 News feed

THE CRIME   THE TIME

 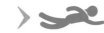

EAT
Burger and chips:
691kcal

DO
Swimming for:
130 minutes

EAT
Glazed doughnut:
242kcal

DO
Crunches for:
88 minutes

EAT
Two pizza slices:
626kcal

DO
Climbing stairs for:
159 minutes

20

The number of grams of protein you need after your evening sweat session to increase new muscle growth while you snooze – the amount in one 200g tub of Fage Total Greek Yoghurt (£1, ocado.com). Getting fitter while you sleep? Perfect.

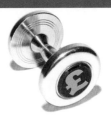

TRAIN TO RESTRAIN

Fancy a splurge? Hit the gym. A moderate intensity session (ie 20-minutes of weights) increases blood flow to the area of the brain responsible for restraint, a VU University Amsterdam study found .

SCREAM IF YOU WANT TO WORK HARDER

That sweaty bloke doing weights isn't grunting to prove his prowess. A study in the *Journal Of Applied Sport Psychology* showed groans can boost performance. Martial artists did a strength test with and without loud vocalisation and hand strength proved greater when they pumped up the volume. Prepare for stares.

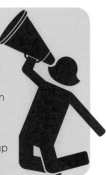

20 MINUTES

THE LENGTH OF TIME YOU NEED TO WORK OUT, THREE TIMES A WEEK, TO REDUCE YOUR CHANCES OF DEVELOPING TYPE 2 DIABETES BY A MASSIVE 33 PERCENT. GET DOWN TO THE GYM AND GIVE US 20!

PART
ONE

FLAT BELLY SECRETS REVEALED

Your new body starts here

Forget your dieting past – the new way to a flat belly starts with putting you back in control, so you'll never feel hungry again

If you've picked up this book, you could probably use a little bit of relationship advice. Hear us out. Most women are in a bad relationship and don't even know it – and the problems have nothing to do with cleaning, cuddling or Sky Sports. It's more fundamental. You want to be in love with each other, but you're stuck in a rut. By now you probably know we're not talking about your man. You're at odds with your own body.

You want to look slim and feel healthy and energised. You want a sexy body that sizzles and the confidence that comes with it. But your body appears to settle for something less. No matter how many diets you try or hours you spend at the gym, nothing changes. Maybe you make a few sacrifices to improve the situation. You eat less, yet still gain weight; buy a gym membership, but see no returns. Maybe you even avoid the foods you love and still get no results.

You're stuck. But unlike a bad boyfriend, you can't break up with your body. It's truly for better or worse. But contrary to what you might think, your body doesn't want a complicated relationship. It wants to be lean, fit, and happy. And your metabolism isn't plotting against you to pack on the pounds. You don't have to settle for anything less than your leanest, sexiest body ever. We're here to make that happen.

Forget past failures and frustrations – that's all about to change. *Flat Belly Workouts* has a few simple steps that will change your relationship with your body for good and unlock the real you. We know all women can be toned, sexy, and confident – without making dramatic sacrifices. And in a matter of weeks, you'll have the body to prove it.

WEIGHT-LOSS TRUTHS

You're probably wondering how this time will be any different. You've tried the diets, done the exercises, and worked hard. You definitely don't have an issue with effort, so maybe you assume that your body is flawed. Maybe you've watched your friends lose weight while you struggle. And there's no shortage of celebs who flaunt their bodies on a weekly basis in magazines and on TV.

Naturally, you might blame yourself for being unable to banish your belly. You know that exercise works. And eating healthy must do something. In fact, you've probably even experienced some success yourself,

> *Flat Belly Workouts* is a proven plan based on information provided by the best experts

say around every January. You start a new programme and things seem great.

But at some point, your regime spirals out of control. You cave to a craving, which starts a downward cycle of bad eating habits. In order to compensate for your struggles, you become desperate to add more "calorie-

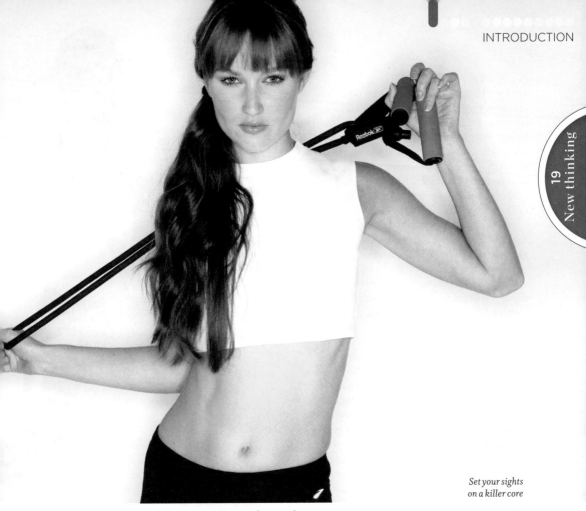

*Set your sights
on a killer core*

burning" cardio, but your body doesn't change. The scales move in the wrong direction. You continue to exercise more and eat less, and still see no difference. What's the problem?

Bad genetics? It's possible. Troubled thyroid? It happens. But more likely, you've yet to tap into the natural mechanisms that help your body burn fat fast.

You see, your body actually is designed to incinerate the chub that covers your sexy abs, firm bum, and lean legs. But the problem is that you've been fed a steady diet of misinformation about what your body needs to look its best. In fact radical, dramatic steps are the last thing your body needs. Sure, those crash diets might provide short-term joy – like a sweet summer fling. But those are usually temporary and end up causing you heartache. You need something more stable.

Flat Belly Workouts is a proven plan based on the information provided by the best fitness and nutrition experts and the latest research. You know what we discovered? If you treat yourself right and follow a few simple guidelines, you can literally switch your body into a fitter, healthier mode – it will burn more calories, build more muscle, and look 10 or even 20 years younger.

The best part: you'll be eating foods that you never thought would be in a diet. You can drink wine without worrying about how many calories are in a glass. You can even indulge in dessert and still flatten your belly. In fact, Greek scientists found that those who don't eat dessert on a healthy eating plan are more likely to gain weight. We've done the research, all you need to do is keep reading and find out how to apply it to your life.

NEW PLAN, NEW YOU

Fit, toned bodies don't come from pills. Or drinks. Or miracle slimming bodysuits. If they did, we'd all look the way we want (and have a more questionable fashion selection than Lady Gaga). And we wouldn't have research, published recently in the *Lancet*, that predicts 43% of British women will be obese by 2030. Do you want to be a statistic or the one who bucks the trend?

We can tell you that exercise and diet work. Extreme behaviours are not the solution. Let's go back to the 1980s. That's when dietary fat was identified as the root of all evil and cardio was elevated to the best form of exercise. Next thing you knew, everyone was gorging on fat-free foods and going on slow jogs.

Fast-forward 30 years and those decades of eating fat-free, sugar-loaded foods have expanded our tummies. And long-slow cardio results in – you guessed it – long, slow weight loss. In a Purdue University study, rats that consumed a mix of low-fat diet crisps plus high-fat crisps gained significantly more fat than rats that only consumed high-fat crisps. It's thought not only did the added sugars add to weight gain, but the low-fat foods failed to dampen hunger signals, tempting the rats to eat more. In addition, Louisiana State University researchers found the average number of calories burned during exercise dropped by 100 calories during the past 20 years, even though people were spending more time in the gym. So it should come as no surprise that the prevailing "best" approach to fat loss resulted in spiralling obesity rates.

We've learned a lot, but people are still relying on old info. It's time to turn the page, debunk myths, and set the record straight: you can have flat, toned belly. Here's why:

YOU HAVE MORE CONTROL

Most fitness plans are inflexible. They are based on a preset routine that doesn't consider your lifestyle. Work, family, friends, and other obligations can make eating healthy and exercising difficult. So much so, according to the Centers for Disease Control

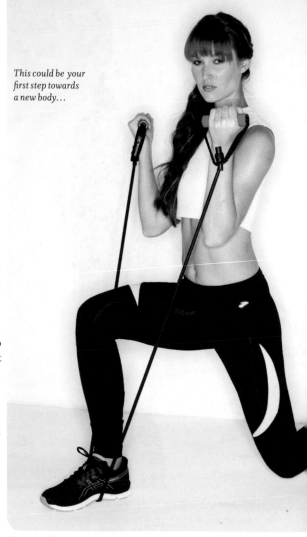

This could be your first step towards a new body…

and Prevention, that people who turn these lifestyle tendencies into excuses were up to 76 percent less likely to lose weight than those who figured out ways around them. In other words: you need to find techniques that won't result in failure, or else you're destined to eventually stop trying.

Flat Belly Workouts works because you can create your own schedule. We empower you to choose how many meals you want to eat, the days you want to exercise, and when you want to escape for a savory dessert or a night out with the girls.

- **You want to eat six meals a day? Go for it**
- **Your schedule won't allow you to eat snacks? Just have three big meals.**

- **You don't have an hour to exercise? No worries, we have body-shaping workouts that will take 20 minutes or less.**

This is the first programme that takes into consideration your priorities and offers the tips you need to look your best.

YOU HAVE MORE FREEDOM

You want to know the real diet secret? Build your plan around foods you love! Let's be realistic: if the only things you eat are brownies and ice cream, you might have to adjust your plan (for the sake of your health most of all!). For everyone else, we insist you keep your favourite foods as part of your diet. The truth is, the negativity surrounding most foods is inaccurate. You can eat white rice and white bread and still lose weight. Pasta doesn't trigger any fat receptors that cause cellulite. And gym sessions do not have to last hours for you to look good in your leggings.

We'll teach you how to load up – the right way – on the food your body craves. You'll be eating what you like, along with what you need, and have more energy and faster fat loss. It's designed to guarantee that you never become tired of what you're eating. By knowing what you can eat – rather than

will teach you how to upgrade your workout to the most efficient plan ever created. You'll learn that weight lifting will not make your muscles look bulky. And how adding just three days of resistance training per week is enough to help you eat less and turn your body into a fat-burning machine 24 hours a day, 7 days a week.

YOUR FIT LIFE STARTS HERE

You'd think that a successful diet and exercise plan would be easy to find. After all, we have more information at our disposal than ever before. But all that information creates a different problem: misinformation – lots of it. That's why you've found yourself struggling to find the solution. Not anymore. We've done the work for you. We've talked to the best experts, read all of the research, and found the best way to get real results.

We've debunked the biggest diet myths, so you'll never veer off track with your eating or exercise. The inspirational recipes in Chapter Three will make every trip to the grocery store an enjoyable experience. We've even included the most pressing concerns and issues that readers have sent directly to *Women's Health* and included them in the book. It's like having your own personal diet coach answering all of your questions – without the ridiculous cost.

We know that living healthy can seem difficult and many people struggle with their weight, whether it's dropping 100 pounds or trimming the last 10. But no matter who you are or where you're starting from, this book is for you. We put our brand behind this title because we know it'll work, using the same winning formula found in the pages of *Women's Health*.

Trust us when we say you'll be more than pleased. You'll eat better, exercise smarter, improve your sex life, and see changes to your overall health. It's the total package. Best of all? When you look in the mirror you'll think, It's good to be me.

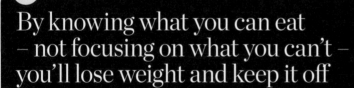

> By knowing what you can eat – not focusing on what you can't – you'll lose weight and keep it off

focusing on what you can't – you'll discover the endless meals that can help you lose weight and keep it off.

YOU HAVE A PROVEN FORMULA

You can't out-exercise a bad diet. That's the most important rule of any successful plan. But a great diet without an exercise plan is incomplete. Your body needs to be active.

But you need to do more than just use the stairs at your office to blast cellulite and make your body sizzle. *Flat Belly Workouts*

Chapter One

A flat belly for life

FIFTEEN LIFESTYLE TWEAKS THAT WILL MELT FLAB AND TONE YOUR BODY

There's one fitness target that's universally understood: a flat belly. No matter how you look at it, a lean, toned midriff represents good health, a fit body and sex appeal. But sometimes it feels like flat abs are like the perfect man: you want to believe they exist, somehow they always seem to elude you. You might even start making excuses: bad genetics, a hectic work schedule, Ben & Jerry's Chunky Monkey ice cream. You can let these excuses get the better of you – or you can take control of your destiny. It's easier than you think! Just like finding the perfect partner, perfect abs are possible once you stop searching so hard for the perfect answer.

You might be trying too hard and overthinking the process. Too many diets and too much exercise have resulted in information overload. It's time to change all of that. Having a great body isn't about sacrifices. It's about understanding how tiny daily changes result in unbelievable transformations. We've seen the fat become thin, mothers who look great in bikinis, and women who eat, drink and still shrink.

Okay, so some women do seem to be born with a great figure and naturally flat tummy. It's just as irritating as those born into huge wealth. But you don't have to be rich to make a lot of money, and you don't need to be born with a six-pack to have toned abs and a flat tummy. Anyone – yes, that includes you – can eliminate their belly and uncover their abs.

The process starts by throwing out the misinformation. We're sure you've heard everything by now. Between crunches, planks, weight training, cardio, six-meals-a-day and weight loss supplements, the process can be overwhelming. So it's time to slow down, hit the refresh button, and take a new, no-nonsense approach to your body. Just by opening this book, you're well on your way. We've filtered out all the bad information, hunted down the top experts, and compiled only the best tips, tricks, and exercises.

The first common myth we'd like to debunk is about your metabolism. No matter how difficult it's been for you to lose weight, your body is not plotting against you. In fact, if you've put on some pounds, your body is working harder to help you get leaner.

Your body burns calories to help you perform all of your daily tasks. This daily maintenance is called your basal metabolic rate (BMR). Everyone has a BMR, but the bigger you are, the faster your metabolism works. Think about that: the more weight you carry, the better your metabolism.

On the surface, it doesn't make sense. After all, skinny people have better metabolisms, right? Well, not exactly. Think

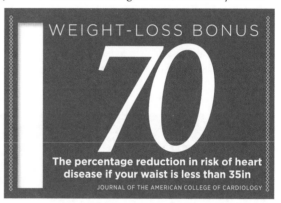

WEIGHT-LOSS BONUS

70

The percentage reduction in risk of heart disease if your waist is less than 35in
JOURNAL OF THE AMERICAN COLLEGE OF CARDIOLOGY

about it another way. Say you have two cars, an Audi and a Rolls Royce. Which needs more fuel? The Rolls does, because it's much larger and has more demands. Your body is no different. The larger you are, the harder your body needs to work and the more calories you burn. Your body wants to be an Audi; you just have to be willing to trade in for a new model.

So how do you become leaner? It's the small things that make the biggest differences. Over time tiny changes add up to a lean body.

Consider this a refreshing outlook on your transformation: your metabolism isn't holding you back, and your body isn't hardwired to look a certain way. You can control your ability to lose weight. Simple, small adjustments to your diet, exercise and other behaviours will make a surprisingly big difference and transform your body.

How easy can it be to see your abs? Here are 15 instant changes you can make that will help your flat belly dreams become a reality.

1. SLEEP MORE AT NIGHT

There's a lot of truth to the term beauty sleep. A Harvard University study of more than 68,000 women found those who slept less than six hours a night weighed 5.4 pounds more and were 15 percent more likely to be overweight than those who got more than seven hours a night. When you sleep less, you experience a drop in the hormone leptin, which controls your appetite, and an increase in the hormone ghrelin – which make you crave food. Those who sleep less eat an average of 220 extra calories per day, say researchers from the University of Chicago. What's more, research in the Netherlands found sleep-deprived women were rated as less attractive and less healthy looking. **Quick Fix #1** Want to eat less and look better? Aim for eight hours a night and don't allow yourself to sleep for less than seven.

Lifting heavy weights can increase your metabolism by 8%, so you'll burn more fat even in your sleep

2. SNACK SMARTER

Snacks are a healthy part of any diet. But, Purdue University researchers say the biggest problem for our weight is that snacks have become meals, and meals have become feasts. In the last 30 years, snack sizes have increased from 360 to 580 calories. That's a whopping 220 extra calories per snack. That number might seem innocent enough in isolation, but so does online shopping. Just as your credit card bill can skyrocket during a few sessions of retail therapy, so can your waistline. In just two weeks, your oversized healthy snacks can contribute to an extra pound of fat. **Quick Fix #2** Enjoy your food, but do it wisely. The lean, nutritious snacks in the meal plan will help you crush your cravings and whittle down your waist.

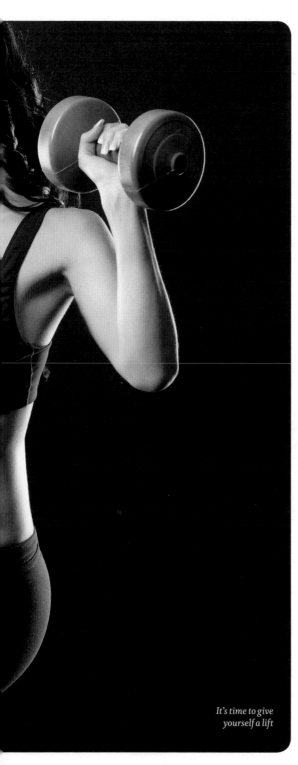

It's time to give yourself a lift

3. EAT MORE, DRINK LESS

Want to instantly drop a dress size? Write down what you eat and drink every day, and then remove all the drinks that aren't water. Now add up the calories. If you're like most women, you'll cut your calories by half, according to the *American Journal of Clinical Nutrition*. Calorie-rich beverages are oftentimes the real culprit behind your weight loss struggles – not your metabolism.
Quick Fix #3 Stick to water, coffee (watch the milk) and tea to help keep your slim-down plan on track. And remember any sugary drink – even fruit juice – should be considered the equivalent of a dessert.

4. LIFT WEIGHTS MORE OFTEN

The calorie tracker on the treadmill might look like a fat-loss genie, but all is not as it seems. That's because the more miles you log, the more efficient your body becomes at running and the fewer calories it burns. In order to ensure your cardio keeps delivering results you need to introduce some variety: some new challenges for your body. Interval training is good, but weight training is even better. Just three days a week of resistance training will offer the metabolic boost you need to slash fat and look hot in any outfit.
Quick Fix #4 Head to the gym three times a week – but don't make the cardio machines your first priority. Instead, use the workouts in this book to fast-track your fat loss.

5. LIFT HEAVIER WEIGHTS

Not only should you lift weights, you should focus on the larger dumbbells. Researchers at Washington University School of Medicine found the more iron you lift, the more fat you burn. It will also increase your sleeping metabolism by 8 percent. So you'll burn more calories even when you're pressing snooze.
Quick Fix #5 When you perform workouts in this book, don't be afraid to use bigger weights as you improve. Each time you reach the goal rep range, increase the weights by 1-2kg. Your hormones will prevent you getting bulky. Heavier weights will only help you sculpt gorgeous, lean muscle.

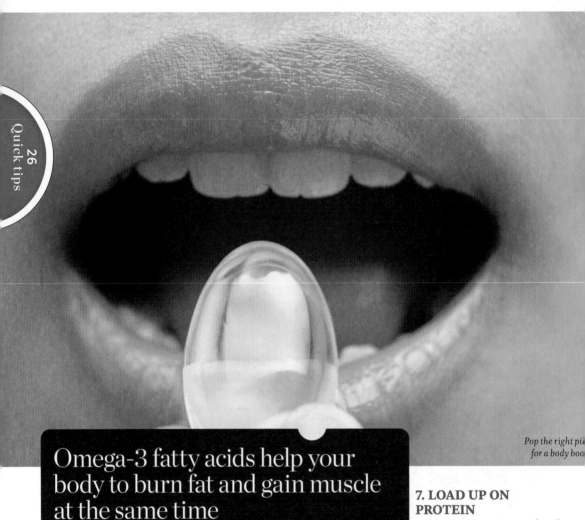

*Pop the right pill
for a body boost*

Omega-3 fatty acids help your body to burn fat and gain muscle at the same time

6. EAT MORE FISH (OIL)

There's nothing fishy about fish oil, especially when it comes to your lean-body goals. Pennsylvania researchers found omega-3 fatty acids might be the secret ingredient to burning fat and gaining muscle at the same time. They also help to lower your cortisol levels – the stress hormone your body produces that makes it more likely you'll store fat and less likely you'll add lean muscle.

Quick Fix #6 Simply make sure you get some oily fish into your diet each day. Salmon, mackerel and sardines are all excellent sources. Or just pop a supplement.

7. LOAD UP ON PROTEIN

Every time you eat a meal and don't consume protein, you're telling your body not to tighten your tummy. Here's why: when you eat other foods – especially carbs – you stimulate insulin, which spikes blood sugar and makes it easier for you to pack on pounds. Even so-called "innocent" foods like fruit can be dangerous. But protein is your solution. It controls blood sugar, reduces hunger and burns more calories during the digestion process so you can stay lean and fit and still enjoy your favourite foods.

Quick Fix #7 Carbohydrates are not bad. But when you eat them alone, they can sabotage your waistline. So always include some protein and you'll drop sizes and stress.

8. DON'T FEAR THE FAT

Eating fat makes you slim. The Institute of Medicine recommends fatty foods make up 20 to 35 percent of your total calories. This, of course, isn't an invitation to head over to the nearest fast-food joint. The fats you want in your diet are saturated fats – from milk, red meat and pork – and monounsaturated fats (MUFAs) like nuts, avocados and oils.

A report published in the *British Journal of Nutrition* found that a MUFA-rich diet helped people lose weight and body fat without changing their calorie intakes. Another report found a breakfast high in MUFAs could boost calorie burn for five hours after you eat.

Quick Fix #8 Fat is your friend. As long as you are staying away from fried foods, trans fats, and partially hydrogenated oils, the healthy fats you eat will make you leaner. Still not sure what to eat? Here are five fatty foods that are good for your body: beef, pork, eggs, sour cream, cheese. Find more delicious foods that slim you down in Chapter Three

9. EAT REAL FOODS

Despite their low-calorie, low-carb, or low-fat claims, "diet" foods might be the worst option if you're trying to lose weight. The reason is simple: diet foods try to trick your brain. They provide you with the flavour of a high-calorie meal without all the calories but are filled with chemicals, artificial sweeteners, and preservatives. Unfortunately, your brain isn't fooled and craves more food, so you overeat. Diet foods are usually devoid of nutritional benefits, so not only do you gain weight, you also deprive your body of the nutrients that protect your general health. Even worse, diet drinks and artificial sugars may increase your risk of metabolic syndrome, which includes higher levels of belly fat, blood sugar, and cholesterol, according to scientists at the University of Minnesota.

Quick Fix #9 Stick to whole, unprocessed foods. As a general guideline, try to shop around your supermarket's perimeter. That's where you'll find more fresh produce. For some of the best foods you'll for your trolley turn to Supermarket sweep on page 64.

10. ENJOY YOUR FOOD

It's not just what you eat – the way you eat might be the best way to curb your hunger. Eating fast makes you gain weight. Japanese researchers found that people who ate faster gained more weight than those who didn't. But if you want to flip the switch on your insatiable appetite, all you need to do is slow down and enjoy. It takes your stomach about 20 minutes to process food and then signal to your brain that you're full. The slower approach will not only leave you more satisfied, but will also help you eat less food, say University of Rhode Island researchers.

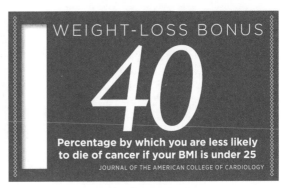

WEIGHT-LOSS BONUS

40

Percentage by which you are less likely to die of cancer if your BMI is under 25

JOURNAL OF THE AMERICAN COLLEGE OF CARDIOLOGY

Quick Fix #10 We don't expect you to bring a timer to your meals, so instead focus on how much you chew your food. Chewing releases more flavour to your tastebuds, which will make all of your meals more enjoyable.

11. WORRY LESS, EAT LESS

Take a deep breath before you head into the kitchen to cook your next meal. As you know, the more stressed-out you are, the more comfort food you crave. This is because stress activates ghrelin, a hormone that makes you feel hungry. The result: you don't achieve satisfaction from your meal, which leaves you craving more food.

Quick Fix #11 The stress in your body is like a light switch: it turns on and off very easily. Simply find a distraction that calms you down and within 5 to 10 minutes, your stress levels will decrease so you can enjoy your meal, without going back for more.

27 Quick tips

12. ENJOY DESSERT

Go ahead, treat yourself – keep it small and frequent. When you're trying to lose weight, the worst thing you can do is ban indulgences. German researchers discovered that this mentality makes it harder to stick to a plan and more likely to pack on the pounds. A more effective approach is one that allows you to satisfy your cravings in controlled portions. Recent research from the University of

WEIGHT-LOSS BONUS

400

Percentage reduction in your stroke risk if your waist is less than 35in

UNIVERSITY OF HEIDELBERG

Alabama found that when overweight women ate small desserts four times a week, they lost 9 more pounds than those who enjoyed a larger splurge whenever they wanted. The small sweets provide the psychological edge that allows you to stay motivated.

Quick Fix #12 Within any diet, 10 to 20 percent of your calories can be a little treat, says nutritionist Alan Aragon. The key is watching the portion size, so that a cup of ice cream doesn't turn into an entire bowl. There are plenty more sweet treats you can enjoy guilt-free in the meal planner from page 50.

13. EAT WITH YOUR GYM CREW

People who work out together should dine together. Eating with those who have a similar goal helps you lose pounds faster, according to a study in the journal *Obesity*. When you're with other people who are trying to lose weight, the social expectation creates different attitudes (for example, you won't have to worry that everyone will be ordering cake for dessert). It's like weight loss osmosis. The good intentions of your fellow eaters rub off on you, and it makes the entire process easier.

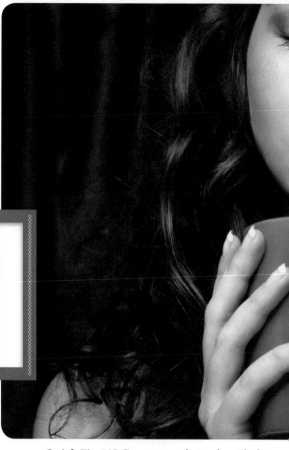

Quick Fix #13 Go out to eat but only with the right crowd! Try to make plans with buddies on a similar track to weight-loss success. Reward yourself with a trip to a fun new restaurant, with those who will encourage you to make the right menu choices.

14. SHAKE UP YOUR DIET

The stuff you see in the window of your local Holland & Barrett isn't just for jocks or serious weight lifters. Those big tubs of protein powder can actually help you flatten your belly. While the appearance might be intimidating, it's exactly what your body needs: an efficient source of protein that is low in calories, helps maintain your hard-earned lean muscle, and helps you lose more fat. The best kind of protein is whey. According to a study in the *Journal of Nutrition*, participants who took whey protein for 23 weeks had less body fat and a smaller waist than those who consumed soy protein.

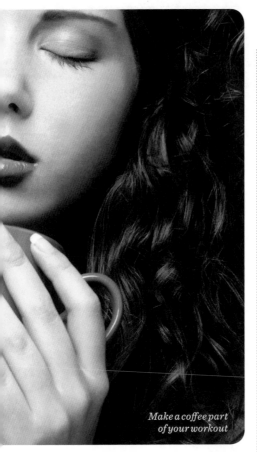

*Make a coffee part
of your workout*

15. WAKE UP TO COFFEE

This might come as a surprise, but the least beneficial aspect of your morning cup of coffee is its ability to provide a sudden jolt and make you more alert. When it comes to improving your health, there are few foods or drinks that offer more universal benefits. The jack-of-all-trades has been shown to improve your workouts by allowing you to push longer and harder and fight off fatigue. But that's just scratching the surface.

Coffee contains more antioxidants than most fruits and vegetables, helping you fight ageing. Harvard researchers also found the magical bean can lower the likelihood of depression by triggering neurotransmitters in your brain that elevate your mood. What's more, women who drink coffee daily reduce their risk of skin cancer by 20 percent. To top it all off, research in the *Archives of Internal Medicine* shows that daily coffee consumption decreases the likelihood of type 2 diabetes, and the American Heart Association reported that coffee reduces the risk of having a stroke by up to 25 percent. All of which is to say, the smartest – and healthiest – way to wake up is with some coffee in your cup.

Quick Fix #15 Don't feel limited to just one morning coffee. Harvard researchers found the sweet spot is two to three cups for the most benefits, and the American Heart Association noted that five cups of coffee can still help your health. If you don't like the buzz, you can still gain all the positives of coffee in the decaf version.

In fact, dieters who included whey protein in their eating plan doubled their fat loss compared to those who ate the same number

Coffee improves your workouts by allowing you to push longer and harder and fight off fatigue

of calories but didn't drink any shakes. Consider protein powder the little bit of extra magic that will finally reveal your abs.

Quick Fix #14 Include a whey protein shake once a day or at least a few times a week. But don't feel you can only have a shake before or after your workout. You can also substitute a breakfast for a shake. Just make them a secondary option to whole foods. You'll find some great shake recipes in Chapter Three.

If these changes seem too easy, it's because having the body you've always wanted isn't as unrealistic as you thought. The real key to a successful diet and exercise plan is cracking the consistency code. You'll eat more, curb hunger, and start whittling your waist down to a sexy, slim silhouette. Forget expensive personal trainers and controlling nutritionists. Let *Flat Belly Workouts* be your coach. Your life-changing journey begins here.

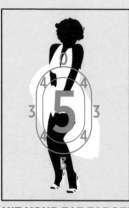

HIT YOUR FAT TARGET

Pot belly ------------------- = 5
Bingo wings --------------- = 4
Cankles --------------------- = 3
Boobs ----------------------- = 0

	Number of hits	Fat value
5		
4		
3		
0		
Fail		
Totals		

Scorer's final weight _____

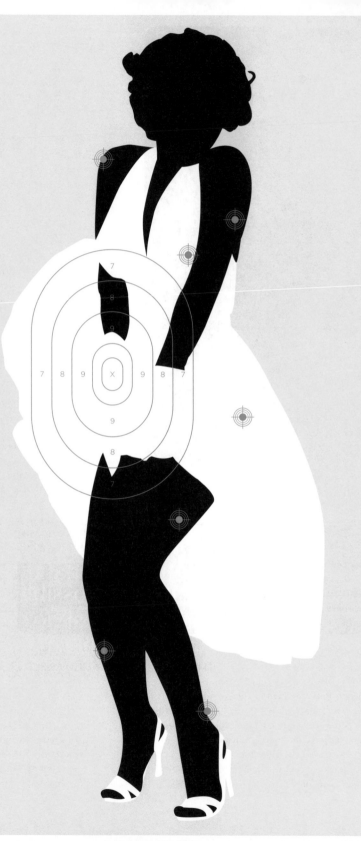

Can you choose where you lose?

It's the sod's law of weight loss: fat comes off the places you don't want instead of the places you do. But new science means all that could be about to change

If you've ever been on a diet, you'll know this story well. Woman restricts calories. She trains like an Olympic athlete. She applies lotions promising 'slimmer thighs and a tighter behind' while submitting her body to massages and machines that profess to blast fat and target bumps and lumps. And yet – after all that effort, all that money – the one place she wanted to drop a few kilos (thighs/bum/insert appropriate body part) she can't.

We have all been told how fat works. Essentially, if the number of calories in beats calories out, you put on weight. But an increasing number of academics and those on the forefront of weight-loss research are beginning to agree that hormones may play a greater part than was once thought when it comes to how and where we store fat. Well, what does that mean for us and virtually every other woman on the planet who's subscribed to the multi-billion pound diet industry at some point? It means this: that at last, we may be able to wage a direct weight-loss assault on the areas we want.

But let's rewind a bit first. A 2008 paper in the *British Journal of Nutrition* suggested that women generally have a larger proportion of body mass as fat, and are more likely to deposit fat subcutaneously (that's a fancy way of saying under the skin) and on their lower half, than men. So we have always accepted that men will have bellies while women will always be saddled with saddlebags and thighs. However, it turns out that it may be possible to target excessive fat in particular areas by realigning hormonal imbalances, says nutritionist Max Tomlinson, author of *Target Your Fat Spots*, who insists "hormones exert a powerful influence on body fat distribution."

We've known for a long time that there's a relationship between hormones and body shape. "Remember your teenage years?" asks Richard Ross, endocrinology lecturer at Sheffield University. "You can't really tell much difference between boys and girls, in terms of body composition, before puberty. At puberty, boys' testosterone switches on and they grow taller and get bigger muscles whereas girls' ovaries switch on, releasing oestrogen and they get breasts and buttocks." Not to mention spots, PMS and inexplicable crushes on their geography teachers.

> It may be possible to target fat by making lifestyle choices that help to realign hormone imbalances

THE BODY'S SIGNATURE

Charles Poliquin is a Canadian strength coach, who over the past few years has caused quite a storm with his Biosignature Modulation Method. He believes you can take an individual's hormonal blueprint (their "biosignature") by taking fat measurements in 12 specific sites on the body using callipers. The data is then used to investigate where hormones are out of whack. Then, believes Poliquin, you can use nutrition, supplements and strength training to realign hormonal imbalances and target individual "fat spots".

If it sounds radical, it is. And Poliquin is not without his critics. While Olympic athletes and even Hollywood stars are said to have adopted his revolutionary approach to training and weight loss, (Superman Henry Cavill's arms were said to be targeted with Poliquin's programme – and have you seen them lately?) there are others who are understandably sceptical.

Skin scientist Peter Roberts, who has previously worked as a national commercial business manager for GlaxoSmithKline and now runs SkinMed, has done extensive academic research into the concept of Biosignature. Yet he remains unconvinced: "There's very little clinical evidence, although there is lots of anecdotal evidence [to suggest Poliquin's method works]. I don't really believe hormones determine whether you lose fat from your bottom or anywhere else. In fact, I'd say if you ran some hormone tests on these people you'd probably find the hormone balance is perfectly normal.'

Poliquin begs to differ. High tricep fat levels, he insists, indicate low testosterone levels. This matches findings from researchers in California, who saw a loss in fat in the upper arm when elevating testosterone to above normal levels in healthy young men.

And before you go thinking, "Well, that's all about men, but what about me?", hold on "Testosterone is produced by both sexes," says Tomlinson. "That means if you have excessive fat on your triceps you may have low levels of testosterone."

Richard Ross agrees: "Androgens [male hormones like testosterone] do burn off body fat both intra-abdominal and subcutaneous areas. If you have an increase in intra-abdominal fat (ie a big tummy) that could be indicative of cortisol excess, growth hormone deficiency and in men it may be associated with testosterone deficiency."

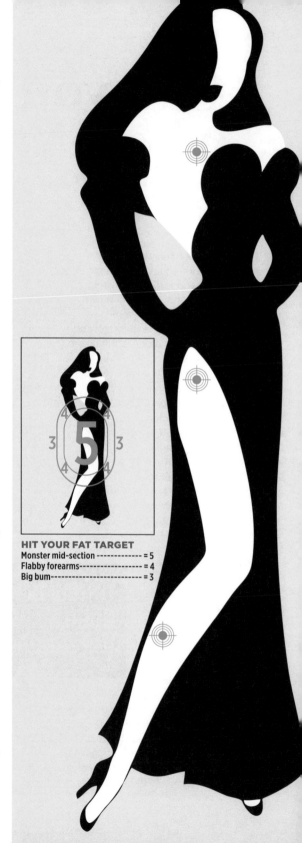

HIT YOUR FAT TARGET
Monster mid-section ------------- = 5
Flabby forearms------------------ = 4
Big bum------------------------- = 3

He also clarifies the link between the thyroid hormone thyroxin and fat gain: "Thyroxin is important for your metabolic rate. So if you have a deficiency in thyroid hormones, you tend to put on fat and find it difficult to lose. And if you have excessive thyroid hormones you burn off fat and muscle."

But Poliquin's analysis takes it a step further and suggests thyroid hormone imbalance is related to upper back fat. Tomlinson, agrees. "Hypothyroidism (low thyroid function) can cause fat deposits around the bra area as well as overall weight gain. No to mention fatigue, depression, constipation and poor concentration." Fun times.

Fat around the stomach area, he also suggests, has a direct correlation with stress hormones. "Stomach fat is a sign of adrenal problems and, more specifically, of over-production of the stress hormone cortisol. Medium to long-term stress elevates cortisol levels, which leads to raised blood sugars and the eventual deposition of blood sugars on the abdomen as fat." So you can blame your boss for that pot belly.

Recent science backs this up: a study published in the *Journal of Psychosomatic Medicine* charted the results when 59 healthy, premenopausal women were exposed to three laboratory stress sessions and one rest session over four days. The 29 of those women who had a high waist to hip ratio (ie held more fat in that area) regarded the challenges as more threatening, performed worse and – lo and behold – secreted significantly more cortisol than the 30 (leaner) women with a low waist to hip ratio. The study's conclusion? Central fat distribution is related to greater psychological vulnerability to stress and cortisol reactivity.

> Stomach fat is a sign of an adrenal problem and the over-production of the stress hormone cortisol

THE ROLE OF TOXINS

According to a study in the scientific journal *Obesity*, stomach fat can also be related to environmental factors. It found having high levels of the environmental toxin PCB (a man-made organic compound used in industry until it was mostly banned in

33
Target fat

Q IS EXERCISE MAKING MY STOMACH FAT?

A You'll probably have heard a little bit about this. No reason to cancel the Zumba class just yet, however. Here's what the deal is: a study by the University of New South Wales found that doing cardio for longer than 45 minutes at a time could increase fat held around the belly. 'If you run for longer than 45 minutes, it's thought that the body releases cortisol in response to the stress of running, which in turn slows your thyroid down,' says nutritionist Max Tomlinson. What's more, the same study, published in the *Journal of Obesity* showed that while the effect of regular aerobic exercise on body fat is negligible, research on HIIE (high intensity intermittent exercise) indicates that it may be more effective at reducing subcutaneous and abdominal body fat than other types of exercise. But there's no need to look far for a programme that follows these rules. The workouts in this book are quick and intense: fat-burning gold.

1986, but which is still found in animals, particularly non grass-fed, and fish) was linked to a high proportion of fat in the abdomen. "These findings may indicate that PCB189, which was also related to developing diabetes, may be of significance in how fat is stored in the body," says Monica Lind, the study's author and associate professor in environmental medicine at the Section for Occupational and Environmental Medicine. Similarly, research published in the US has linked a chemical found in non-stick pans and water-resistant fabrics to an under-functioning thyroid. So, what's a girl to do?

"What I prescribe is a three-pronged approach that includes targeted exercise and corrective eating, as well as taking specific supplements," says Tomlinson, who adds that we can't get enough vital nutrients from modern foods.

Poliquin also believes in supplements to counteract the effect of ingesting inevitable environmental toxins, suggesting natural supplements such as glycine, vitamin C, selenium and N-acetyl cysteine (NAC).

The UK Food Standards Agency, while agreeing that "PCBs are found at low levels in all foods, including foods that are important sources of nutrients," disagrees: "The Agency's advice is that the benefits of a healthy, balanced diet, outweigh any risks from dioxins and PCBs." So what should we believe? Best to ask someone who's tried it: Katie Dixon first had her Biosignature test done at the start of 2012 and won Britain's strongest woman under 75kg in September of the same year. Dixon was so impressed that she signed up to become a Poliquin practitioner. She was struggling with fat around the hamstrings. Poliquin puts fat

FOUR WAYS TO STABILISE HORMONES

Eat mindfully, add spice, cut the sugar and get plenty of rest to give your body the best shot at regulating hormones and minimise fat gain in unwanted areas

1 SWEET IT OUT
Cut sugars and refined carbohyrates – we're talking simple carbs like sugar, white bread, you know the suspects. They are quickly absorbed into the bloodstream and cause your blood glucose levels to rise sharply and produce elevated insulin levels (which, over time, causes fat deposits around the sides of the stomach). Watch out for hidden sugars in things like baked beans, orange juice, flavoured yoghurts and alcohol. To help you out, download the GI Monitor app.

2 SPICE IT UP
Add cinnamon to everything: this super-spice can help slow the speed at which food leaves your stomach and glucose enters the bloodstream by up to 35%, according to research published in the *American Journal of Clinical Nutrition*, helping to keep blood sugar levels stable. The more stable your blood sugar, the less likely you are to overproduce insulin, develop insulin resistance and thus lay down tummy fat. How's that for a slimline spice?

3 SLEEP ON IT
When you rest, your body has time to regulate hormones. Promote good sleep by using a blind, not eating anything sugary and not using technology an hour before bed and going to bed and waking up at a similar time every day. Losing just one hour's sleep a night could raise insulin levels in the body, as well as exhaustion-related bad food cravings and skipped gym sessions. Watch your caffeine intake, too, it releases cortisol and keeps you up.

4 MIND FOOD
Start eating mindfully. A recent study in the *Journal of Obesity* found a mindful eating practice (you know, just you, the food, no phone, no computer, no social media, not even a book) was linked to reduced cortisol levels and a decrease in belly fat. To help you out on learning how to eat mindfully, listen to meditation guru Andy Puddicombe's podcast, or download the app Headspace-on-the-go. All together now: Omm...

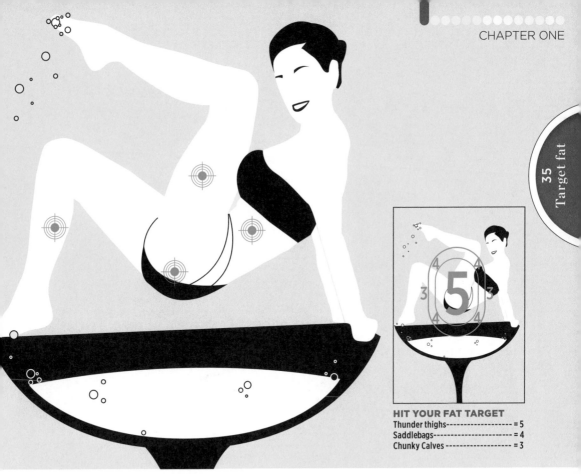

HIT YOUR FAT TARGET
Thunder thighs------------------ = 5
Saddlebags--------------------- = 4
Chunky Calves ------------------ = 3

stored here down to too many toxins in the body. Katie followed a 12-week liver protocol, taking supplements supposed to boost liver function, and says: "After completing it, my hamstring readings were the lowest they'd ever been. Nothing else changed, my diet stayed the same but the supplements helped me strip some of the fat from my legs."

THE ROLE OF VITAMINS

The problem remains that we don't know for sure whether these changes are definitely the result of supplementation (they could be psychosomatic, for example). Even Poliquin devotees, like Dixon's trainer, James Smith of Elite Bodyworks, often believe that supplements should be handled with care. "For most women, there will be a big improvement in hamstring fat levels with an increase in fibre, green vegetables and the removal of sugar from the diet," he

says. "I'd try to get everything else on track before we look at supplementation. Nobody takes enough omega-3s, nobody produces enough magnesium or zinc; I'd suggest those whether you're an elite athlete or a coach potato. A bit of vitamin B might help, too. But the lifestyle changes, such as eating the right things at the right time and recovering effectively from training sessions, are the most important things in losing fat."

In fact, he insists that sleep is the unsung hero when it comes to getting rid of fat in those stubborn areas: "Sleep is one of the most powerful ways your body regulates hormones."

So what (and who) can we believe for sure? It's still an ongoing argument but for now we do know that the four study-backed tips, left, will go some way to targeting your belly. And that's not a bad place to start, right?

Chapter Two

Questions and answers

EXPERTS ANSWER THE MOST-ASKED
WEIGHT-LOSS QUESTIONS FROM
WOMEN'S HEALTH READERS

Whats the fastest way for me to lose weight?" It's the one question that is asked repeatedly at *Women's Health*, and for good reason. For many women, the answer seems like a puzzle. Whether you're an apple or a pear, it can feel very frustrating trying to find the right plan for you. But no matter which fruit you identify with, the right plan should empower you to successfully drop excess weight, look great in your clothes, and feel confident about your appearance.

The truth is, there's no one "fastest" way. It really depends on your lifestyle, food preferences, and how often you make health a priority. The simple answer is a combination of diet and exercise, but that's the type of answer that has frustrated you in the past.

Here's what you need to know for your future: you deserve to lose weight. You work hard, and you should reap the rewards. So savour this answer: anyone can eliminate their belly and transform their body. Even better? The road isn't as bumpy as you think, but it does require a few changes. To put you on a fast track to a flatter belly, we posed the most common weight-loss questions to the *Women's Health* fitness and nutrition experts. They're here to eliminate your confusion, end your frustration, and provide a perfect road map to looking and feeling better now. These aren't just answers – they are the secrets you need to banish your former body and replace it with the one you've always wanted.

Q I'm losing pounds but not inches. What's wrong?

A Usually this means you're not weight training or eating enough protein, says nutritionist Alan Aragon, who has worked with Olympic athletes. Doing both is the key to eliminating fat and building muscle – as opposed to just losing weight. That's the real key to looking like you have a new body, rather than just seeing a different number on the scales. Resistance training burns calories during your sessions and stimulates your metabolism afterwards. Make sure you get enough protein after a workout by adding

either 170g of meat or 2 scoops of protein powder; each option yields about 40g protein.

Q I thought protein shakes were just for bulky men

A No way! Don't be fooled by the big-muscle guys on protein pots. Women can absolutely benefit from protein shakes, especially if they have a tough time hitting their protein requirement through regular foods. There's nothing sex-specific about protein shakes – but I bet you'll feel a whole lot sexier after incorporating them into your plan and seeing the results you get.

Q How often do I need to exercise to lose fat?

A Surprisingly you don't need to exercise to lose fat. You can shed your unwanted pounds simly by eating fewer calories than you burn, says Aragon.

However, if you avoid exercise, you won't retain as much muscle, which means it'll be harder for you eliminate your muffin top and have a flat, sexy tummy. You can lose weight

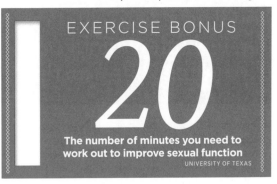

EXERCISE BONUS

20

The number of minutes you need to work out to improve sexual function
UNIVERSITY OF TEXAS

without exercise, but if you don't retain or build muscle, your metabolism won't be as efficient, which means you'll have to eat even less food to see the same results.

So how much exercise should be done to help with fat loss? Take note, gym haters, it's really not that huge of a commitment. With just 30 minutes a day, three days a week, you can eat the foods you want and fast-track your weight loss. You'll find all the exercises you need in this book, starting in Chapter Four.

Q **I always gorge after a workout. Bad habit?**

A Post-workout is actually the best time to have the largest meal of your day – as long as it's a reasonable size and not a full-on gorge. That's because you've just reduced your body's fuel reserves, and food can help aid your recovery. Also, when your body is in a recovery state, incoming calories stand a better chance of being absorbed by muscle tissue instead of being stored as fat.

If your goal is to curb uncontrollable hunger after a workout, make sure you're filling up on beef, poultry, or fish. Solid foods are more filling than liquid foods, and protein is the most filling. Pair some of that meat with high-fibre carbs, such as beans, which can also help you feel fuller faster, and for longer.

Q **Do I need to count calories to lose weight?**

A Counting calories is a way of staying consistent with an eating plan that will allow you to lose weight, says Aragon. But

with more substantial meals less frequently. Whether you prefer an even split of calories over six meals or three larger meals you should always plan healthy snacks. Everyone gets peckish now and then. If you've got a bag of nuts to hand you won't see your weight-loss derailed by an afternoon a chocolate binge.

Q **Can I have dairy and still lose my belly?**

A They myth that high-fat foods make you fatter made dairy a dirty word for many years. In fact, researchers from the University of Tennessee found that milk will help you flatten your belly as its calcium aids digestion. You can even enjoy high-fat cheeses and yogurts if you prefer. The trick is, make sure you don't eat too much. Dairy is generally high in calories, so keep an eye on your portion size – and then, enjoy!

You'll be able to eat more food and feel full without ever expanding your waistline

that doesn't mean you need to do it to be effective. In fact, in this book you'll find a no-calorie counting method that sparks fat loss. The foods in this diet are flexible so that you can choose your meals. But they also focus on foods that are energy dense, such as protein, fruits, vegetables and grains. You'll be able to eat more of these foods and feel full without expanding your waistline. You'll eat better, and you'll be drop pounds, too.

Q **Will eating smaller meals control my hunger?**

A Food is like fashion sense: it's all personal preference. Some people prefer a grazing pattern, while others do well

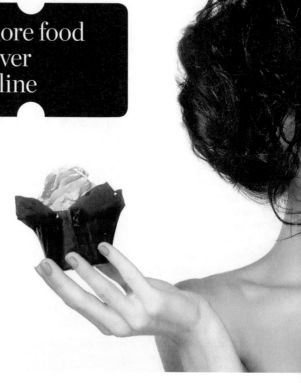

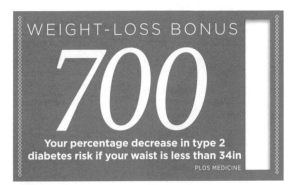

700

Your percentage decrease in type 2 diabetes risk if your waist is less than 34in

PLOS MEDICINE

Q **I don't want to totally cut out carbs, but does that mean I won't lose weight?**

A In a word, no. Your belly is formed by eating too many unused calories. If you overeat, you'll store fat, regardless of where those calories are coming from, says Aragon. As you'll find out, every food is fair game on

Have your cake… but eat the apple first

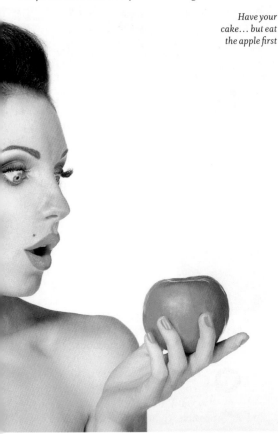

the eating plan you'll use in this book. That said, processed carbs – anything that hasn't come straight out of the ground or off a tree – are easier for your body to break down so will turn to fat more quickly. So try to get most of your carbs from fruit and veg, not cake and pasta. If you're imaginative, you can turn even turn veg into a pasta substitute.

Try spaghetti squash, which has almost the same consistency as the traditional Italian dish, but with only a fraction of the calories. (We promise, you will be shocked at how good this tastes). Just cut the squash in half and microwave for 6-8 minutes. Then, use a fork and run it through the squash – from top to bottom – to create spaghetti-like strands. Add a sauce or some veggies or meatballs, serve and enjoy.

39 Q&A

Q **I sit at a desk all day. Is there anything that I can do at work to improve my abs?**

A Get up from your desk as often as you can. A minimum of every half hour, try to at least stand up and stretch, then walk around, walk over to a colleague's desk instead of emailing them, or take a lap around the office, says Aragon. This process is important because it increases your non-exercise activity thermogenesis (NEAT).

Your NEAT plays a big role in the number of calories you burn, so even small movements like fidgeting or tapping your heels can contribute to your overall transformation, although they'll have more of an impact if you do them while standing.

This will also help prevent your desk job from altering your posture, which can play a role in your slowed metabolism (not to mention an aching back!).

Q **I've been told not to eat late, but usually I'm starving after my shift. What should I do?**

A Your body does not process all foods in the same way, so the trick is to avoid fast-digesting, refined carbs like bread and pasta. Your body breaks these down extremely quickly and within a just a few

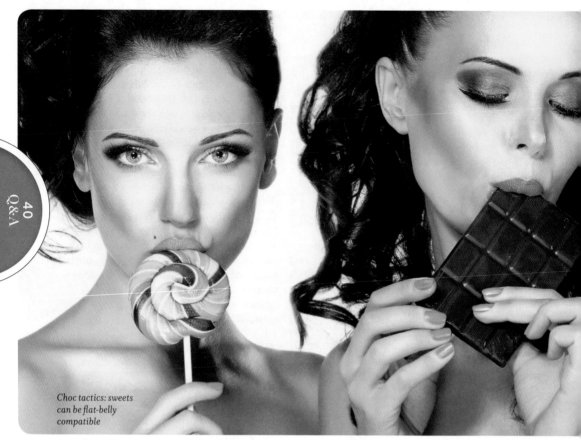

Choc tactics: sweets can be flat-belly compatible

minutes will extract simple sugars (glucose) from them. Glucose is your body's primary energy source, so really great if you're about to do a workout… not so great if you're about to go to bed. That glucose will get stored, some of it in your muscles, but most as fat. Instead make high-protein, high-fat foods your late

> The way most women approach running - long slow jogs- is not an efficient way to blast away fat

night snacks – think meat, cheese and nuts. Protein in these foods will go to muscle building, particularly if you've been working out that day. And the extra time they take to digest means you won't get a huge rush of glucose that your body has to store somewhere (usually your belly, bum and thighs).

Q What are the worst foods for my abs?

A Your focus shouldn't be on what's worst, but instead on what's best. A great diet – like the one in this book – highlights healthy foods that make dropping pounds easy. What matters most for shedding belly fat boils down to calories in versus calories out. It might be tempting to call a certain food, like chocolate, "bad" for your abs. But if it is part of a diet dominated by whole foods, it could actually be "great" for your abs. Small indulgences are often what helps you stick to your plan. Virtually no foods are off-limits as long as they're in small portions.

Q Can I get flat abs without doing any crunches?

A You want to lose belly fat as fast as possible, right? In order to do that, you need exercises that activate the most number of muscle fibres, says Olympic strength coach Eric Cressey. Crunches simply don't cut it. When you perform multi-muscle and multi-joint exercises, you're also working your abs, whether you realise it or not.

This is why movements like squats, deadlifts, lunges, chin-ups and press-ups are so effective. They work the muscles you feel (legs, arms, chest, back, shoulders) and your abs, too. Any workout that incorporates these moves will keep your core working overtime and ensure you get a flat belly in no time.

These compound exercises allow you to do more in less time. They stimulate greater fat loss, and they also carry over to a healthier overall lifestyle. Whether it's picking up a toddler or reaching for a high shelf, compound movements prepare you for lots of everyday challenges.

And a little bit of strength goes a long way in making your life easier, such as preventing nagging issues – like throwing out your back or having sore knees – that occur naturally when you avoid these types of exercises.

Q Won't gaining muscle make me look bulky?

A Weight training can be very deceiving. When you see men lifting huge weights it's easy to assume that's the reason their muscles are popping out of their T-shirts.

But it's tremendously challenging for women to gain muscle like a man, says Cressey. The reason: women have far less testosterone than men, which makes it an uphill battle to add significant muscle mass, let alone enough size to make you look bulky. That alone is enough to not worry about any negative impact of pumping a little iron.

41
Q&A

THREE ABS MYTHS, BUSTED

With so much abs advice out there, it's hard to know what really works. There's a place for almost every type of exercise, but here's how to really make the most of every rep

MYTH #1:
High-rep workouts make your abs grow

REALITY: Your progress will plateau if you do the same exercises, regardless of reps. Intensify your workout by doing more challenging variations of bodyweight exercises and start using weights once they become too easy. Matt McGorry, CFT, a trainer at Peak Performance in New York, recommends the rolling plank. This combo – see page 154 for a full description – forces you to contract your abs for long intervals. Hold each plank for 15 seconds and work up to 60. "But bear in mind, no amount of abs work can take the place of a well-planned diet and a total-body workout," McGorry says.

MYTH #2:
Abs workouts involve a lot of movement

REALITY: Exercises that require steadiness are best. When you bend your spine during crunches or sit-ups, you risk injuring it, says Stuart McGill, PhD, a professor of spine biomechanics at the University of Waterloo in Ontario. You're repeatedly bending the disks in your back, not forcing your abs to resist motion. Exercises that prevent movement are great for building lateral abdominal strength, which is what helps your body stay in form under pressure. McGill suggests the suitcase carry: hold a heavy dumbbell in one hand and walk increasingly long distances. This burns more calories than crunches!

MYTH #3:
Rotational exercises are best for building obliques

REALITY: Rotational exercises don't build obliques well at all, and can harm the spine in some cases. So while exercises like twisting side to side while holding a weight can help you build your obliques, they may not be the best way to build foundational strength. Instead, use heavy compound exercises – like squats and deadlifts – to make your obliques keep your spine aligned. These types of exercises require your body to adjust to uneven stress while your spine is in its neutral position, which further stabilises your core and builds your obliques, as long as you maintain proper form.

Also, putting on major muscle mass is a struggle for many women because it takes a high volume of strength training in combination with lots of extra calories. On this plan, you'll be eating just the right amount of calories and doing just the right amount of reps to achieve long, lean muscles – not a bulky, bodybuilder bod.

Q Isn't running the fastest way to lose weight?

A Running is a great form of exercise, and great for overall cardiovascular health. But the way that most women approach running – with long, slow jogs – is not an efficient way to blast fat, says Cressey.

If running is your preferred form of exercise, then stick to interval training. It has you working at a high level of intensity for short periods of time, followed by quick rest periods. Overall, your cardio workouts will be shorter but much more effective.

Adding lean muscle tone helps you to burn more calories, even when you're not exercising

If you want to shed pounds fast, you'll need to spend the bulk of your exercise time performing resistance training. As we already mentioned, lifting weights won't make you bulky (promise!), but give you great definition and shape. Adding lean muscle tone helps you burn more calories, even when you're not exercising. Bottom line: resistance training doesn't just take body fat off – it keeps it off.

Q Are their any other benefits to lifting weights?

A Of course. You'll improve bone and cardiovascular health, as well as optimising glucose control so your body processes carbs better. Plus, in addition to sculpting your abs, you'll gain definition in

your arms and legs. Imagine slipping on a little black dress and turning heads all night. Can you think of better motivation to pick up a dumbbell? Didn't think so!

Q How do I know what fat is okay to eat?

A There's no need to avoid any particular type of fat, except for partially hydrogenated vegetable oils (trans fats). Recent research shows that even the link between saturated fats and cardiovascular disease may have been overstated. And while you don't want to be gorging on fatty meat every day, the fact is your diet probably doesn't include enough fat. The standard British diet lacks omega-3 fatty acids, found naturally in oily fish such as salmon. The majority of the fats you eat should come from minimally processed foods like lean meat, fish, dairy, vegetables, fruits, nuts, seeds, avocados and olive oil. Not too much of a hardship, eh?

Q Should I take supplements to help define my abs?

A Most fat-loss supplements are a waste of money and some have risks that outweigh any small benefit, says Aragon.

The most potent fat-burning supplements contained caffeine and ephedrine. That combination was banned from the market due to too many reports of adverse, dangerous side effects. The truth is, the actual fat loss caused by any supplement is minor and insignificant in people who are overweight or have a substantial amount of weight to lose, says Aragon. Bottom line: the best and only real way to see your abs is to focus on two things: what you eat and how you exercise.

Q What's the fastest way to jump-start my weight loss when it comes to diet?

A Eat more food. Seriously this will work. But make sure your selections are nutrient-dense foods that will leave you

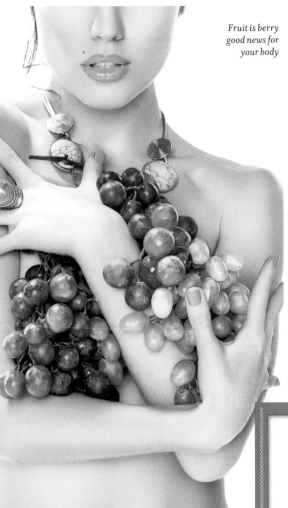

Fruit is berry good news for your body

carbohydrate source of all. These natural foods are not only filled with vitamins and minerals, they're also lower in calories, which means you can eat more without overindulging.

What's more, fruits and vegetables are also loaded with belly-filling fibre that will keep you satisfied longer and fight off your hunger pangs. And the sugar in fruit will satisfy your sweet tooth, without drastically impacting your insulin levels and thus avoiding excess fat storage.

Q Is it okay to have artificial sweeteners?

A This is an area of big debate among nutritionists, but there's no scientific evidence that artificial sweeteners contribute to weight gain. That said, make sure you don't abuse diet fizzy drinks, which are filled with fake sugars, says Aragon. The problem is, fooling your body into thinking it is taking on sugar, while depriving it of the calories it expects, could make you feel hungry soon afterwards and also prime your sweet tooth to crave sugary foods every day.

43
Q&A

WEIGHT-LOSS BONUS

40

Percentage by which you cut your risk of arthritis if your BMI is under 25

UNIVERSITY OF NOTTINGHAM

more satisfied with fewer calories. A great example of this is what's known as carb-swapping, says Aragon.

The process is simple: replace any processed carbohydrate you eat (think white rice, pasta, and bread) with fruits and vegetables. Processed carbs are higher in calories and digested quickly so they don't leave you particularly satisfied. Carbs that have had less refinement, think brown rice and pasta, are better as they are slower to digest, so yield their energy more gradually. But fruits and vegetables are the best

Artificial sweeteners are fine on the odd occasion, but if your diet consists mainly of whole foods, you can enjoy a little sugar every now and then, whether it's artificial or not. Sugar in sensible amounts is a good treat to help keep your weight-loss on track, plus it can give you an energy boost before or after a big workout. So, really, it's best to give the artificial stuff the boot completely and stick to the white stuff.

Chapter Three

Fuel your goals

THE NUTRITION SECRETS THAT WILL POWER YOUR WORKOUTS AND GET YOU THE BODY YOU WANT, FAST

The fix to all of your dieting woes can be solved in three words: stop counting calories. That was the message of a 20-year study on weight loss conducted at the Harvard School of Public Health. The researchers concluded dieters who only focused on how much they ate – rather than the types of foods – were more likely to fail at losing weight.

The reason: counting calories isn't sustainable and causes stress, which increases the likelihood of long-term failure. That's not to say that counting calories doesn't work. It does. It's worth being aware of how much key foods contain so you don't get caught out. But the simple fact is that it's virtually impossible to keep track of your exact calorie intake at every meal, day in, day out. So instead, with the Flat Belly Plan, your goal isn't to minimize how much you eat. It's to make sure you're filling your body with quality foods that will help you lose weight. Knowing what to eat should be simple, not stressful. So, we've devised a series cheats that offer all the benefits of counting calories – without the maths.

If you want to experience success like never before, all you have to do is live by these five mantras. They blast fat, let you enjoy food without guilt, and make you look and feel younger than ever. Say them out loud. Learn them by heart. Pretty soon they'll become as much a part of your daily routine as checking out your hot new reflection in the mirror! The first isn't food related at all. It's a reminder of the workouts around which your nutrition plan will be built:

FLAT-BELLY MANTRA 1
"I WILL NOT BE AFRAID TO LIFT WEIGHTS"

We've said it before, but we can't stress this enough. Running burns calories, but it's not the best way to burn fat. If your goal is to tighten your tummy and firm up your legs and bum, then fat loss – not just lowering the number on the scales – is what matters. And for maximum fat loss, lifting weights is the only way to go.

Scientists at the University of Connecticut found dieters who lifted weights lost nearly 40 percent more fat than those who did only cardio, even though exercise time was the same. Here's why: weight training keeps your internal furnace burning for days after you complete your last rep. Just three sessions a week can reduce your body fat by three percent in 10 weeks – even without changing your diet. It might not seem like much, but that can mean three inches off your waist. What's more, new muscle will help you body burn even more fat. A study in *Medicine & Science in Sports & Exercise* found that after six months of lifting weights just three days a week, metabolism was boosted by seven percent.

Of course, that should be reason enough to pick up a dumbbell. But the benefits of weight training are even sweeter: not only do you have to work out fewer times per week, you also have shorter sessions, because intensity is much more important than duration for eliminating fat. In fact, 12 minutes of intense intervals burns as many calories as 25-30 minutes of constant moderate exertion.

Right now, you might be thinking, "Why run?" If you enjoy it, that's reason enough. Traditional cardio is still good for your body and your heart, and it does burn calories. So if you have time, you can make it a part of your workout routine. In fact, we recommend it. And of course, if you're training for a marathon or are active in sports, your plan

> # Just three sessions of weights per week can knock three inches off your waist in 10 weeks

will require more cardio. But if you're tight on time (and we know you are), then weight training should be your priority. The science proves you don't need much time lifting weights to make big changes to your body. In just 30-45 minutes per workout, you'll get leaner and more toned.

45 Meal plans

FLAT-BELLY MANTRA 2
"I WILL MAKE GREEN MY NEW FAVOURITE COLOUR"

Here's a rule you probably never thought you'd hear suggested in a diet plan: eat as much as you want. But that's exactly what we want you to do with green vegetables. Whether you prefer spinach, broccoli, asparagus or exotic offerings like bok choy and kale, pile your plate high with as many as you like. Vegetables are packed with so many super nutrients that they have been linked to almost every health benefit imaginable – heart health, cancer prevention, a boost in mood and energy, they've even been found to help rev up your sex life.

But the biggest benefit is weight loss. A study in *The American Journal of Clinical Nutrition* found women who included veggies in every meal were able to eat 25 percent more food but lose an additional 3.5 pounds. How? Vegetables are low in calories but they also rev your fat burn because they are full of fibre, which keeps you feeling satisfied, so you're less likely to overeat later.

What's more when it comes to portion control, the similar rules go for fruit, which brings us to the next mantra…

FLAT-BELLY MANTRA 3
"I WILL TRADE EMPTY CALORIES FOR REAL CARBS"

If there's one food group you should avoid on this plan, it's refined sugar. Your fix: eat more fruit. Fruit – nature's sweet reward – provides plenty of carbs for energy, but has less impact on your blood sugar than processed sweets and other carbohydrates. This is crucial to help you avoid the cravings and binges that occur when your blood sugar rises quickly and then

THE TRUTH ABOUT PROCESSED FOODS
Why 'pierce film lid' should never have a place in your meal preparations

Stop us if this sounds familiar: "All calories are equal, so it doesn't matter what I eat." It's a mantra that's older than Barry Humphries, and it's a diet fallacy that drives nutritionists mad.

Processed foods (like cakes and biscuits) that are high in refined carbs and sugars can make you crave more food. As a result, you eat more than you need at your current meal – and the next, say Syracuse University researchers. It's dietary double jeopardy: you eat more than you need, and you don't receive any nutritional benefit.

This is why fruits and vegetables need to make up most of your carbohydrates. They do what food is supposed to – leave you satisfied. These natural sugars don't play tricks on

your mind or your body, and you'll be able to eat without any guilt or the fat to show for it.

Like anything in life, moderation is the key to balance. "You don't need to completely remove processed foods from your diet, but keep them to a maximum of 10 to 15 percent of your daily calories," says nutritionist Dr Alan Aragon. When you eat more than that, you risk creating a diet that doesn't provide you with the vitamins, minerals and nutrients your body needs. While it might not seem that important, research has found that a diet high in processed foods increases your risk for cardiovascular diseases and metabolic syndrome.

What's more, eating processed foods actually

slows down your metabolism, which is why you want to follow our suggested guidelines. Researchers from Pomona College found that meals consisting of processed foods burn significantly fewer calories than a less processed meal. In fact, a 20-year review conducted by the *New England Journal of Medicine* unlocked the reason why so many people gain weight: processed foods.

The researchers found that processed foods – like crisps, biscuits and chips – cause people to gain up to 17 pounds over a 20-year span. If your plan is to eat, drink and still shrink, then replacing the processed snacks in your diet can be the small change that finally helps you have a flat, toned belly.

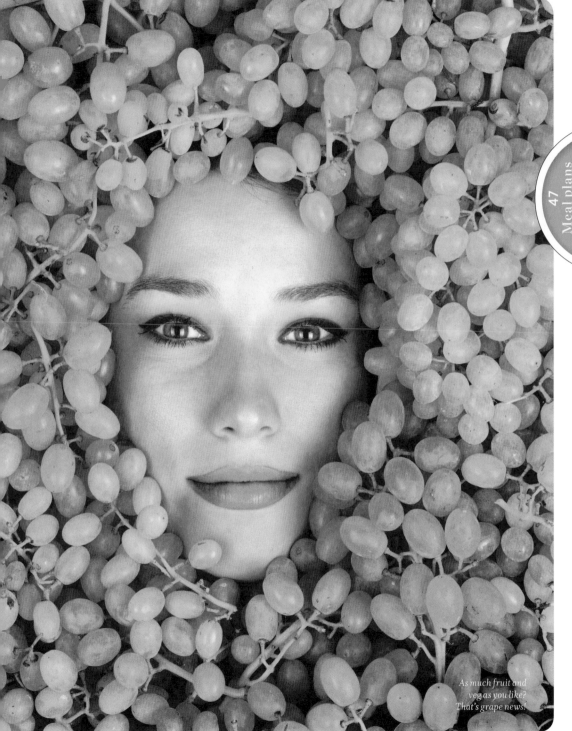

As much fruit and veg as you like? That's grape news!

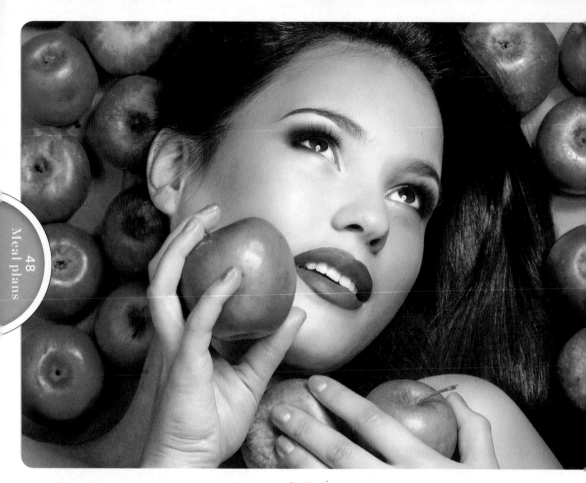

crashes. Ideally, the majority of your carbs will come from fruits. That doesn't mean you won't have grains, beans or other carbs and the occasional treat, but they will be a secondary source. Limit yourself to a couple daily servings of sugars and processed carbs (bread

> The way most women approach running - long slow jogs- is not an efficient way to blast away your fat

and pasta), and consume the rest from fresh produce. You'll soon find you don't even miss sugary snacks. A sweet apple, orange or banana will do the same job. Remember to eat protein regularly, too... you'll never feel full on fruit alone. Which brings us to...

FLAT-BELLY MANTRA 4
"I WILL BECOME BEST FRIENDS WITH PROTEIN"

When it comes to a thinner waist, protein is your best friend. Try to include at least a little bit of protein in every meal and snack. It keeps you feeling full and is less likely to be stored as fat. That's because protein is harder to digest, so you burn more calories just eating it. This process also helps ensure you eat less. A recent study in *Nutrition & Metabolism* found women whose diet was 30 percent protein ate almost 450 calories less per day and lost 11 pounds more than those who ate less protein. British researchers found that emphasising protein in each meal leaves you feeling fuller, accelerates fat loss, and spares your muscle mass, which is key to

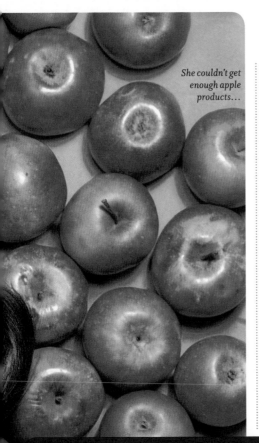

She couldn't get enough apple products…

shedding pounds and revealing your flat belly. So whether it's fish, eggs, yoghurt or cheese, you'll need a constant source of nature's ultimate abs superfood, the plan on the following pages will ensure you get it.

FLAT-BELLY MANTRA 5
"I WILL DRINK LOTS OF WATER"

Dehydration is the enemy of fat burning. If your body doesn't have enough water it won't metabolise fat at peak efficiency. What's more if there is a lack of water coming into your system it will hold onto what it has,causing bloating (water retention). In the meal planners that follow there are no drinks listed, however aim for at least six glasses a day (1.5 litres). Tea counts as hydration. Coffee, however, does not (although it can give you a useful pre-workout boost). Don't take sugar with either. Treat any other drinks with caution. Even seemingly healthy options like orange juice hide large amounts of sugar. And alcohol, while not forbidden, should be for special occasions only. Turn to page 76 to negotiate the booze minefield.

49 | Meal plans

HOW THE FLAT BELLY MEAL PLANNER WORKS
Your eating plan begins on the next page. Here's the thinking behind it

More nutritional information is available to us today than ever before, yet we still can't seem to figure out the most basic question – how often do I need to eat to lose weight? Here's a waist-trimming tip that you might find soothing: the latest research shows that it doesn't really matter how frequently you eat. All that matters is what you eat.

Many modern diet plans suggest five or six evenly sized meals spread throughout the day. This can be somewhat impractical and portion sizes can get out of hand. Instead the Flat Belly Plan you'll find on the following pages

suggests three main meals a day, with healthy snacks in between. Snacking is often a helpful tactic. Too often people on diets try to resist it, meaning that by the time they sit down for their main meal they are famished and end up overeating. Just make sure your snacks are healthy ones (not crisps and chocolate) You'll find plenty of suggestions on the following pages.

If, however, you find that snacking doesn't work for you, eat less often. Overall intake is the bottom line.

You can use the planners on the following pages as you see fit. Either follow them word-for-word, or

use them as inspiration for creating your own healthy menus. The aim of them is to show how it is possible to create a diverse, practical menus day after day and week after week.

The main thing is not to overthink the eating process. As we mentioned earlier, counting calories doesn't work. Eating healthy, natural foods at every meal does. Your body will use foods in the right way as long as you are making sure that most of your foods come from proteins, vegetables, and fruits. Remember, extreme plans don't work! Take control of the situation and your belly will disappear fast.

Week 1

	MONDAY	TUESDAY	WEDNESDAY	THURSDAY	FRIDAY	SATURDAY	SUNDAY
Breakfast	*Yoghurt and Fruit* •245g plain Greek yoghurt •1 handful blueberries •60g granola	*Strawberry-Banana Protein Smoothie* (page 60)	*Mexican Scrambled Eggs* •2 eggs, •Chopped tomatoes, onions, spinach, and peppers •30g grated cheese •100g salsa	*Almond Butter on Toast* •1 slice wholemeal toast •1 tablespoon almond butter •½ pint semi-skimmed milk	*Egg and Cheese Sandwich* •2 eggs scrambled •1 slice of cheese •English muffin, toasted	*Strawberry Protein Pancakes* •1 scoop vanilla protein powder •1 egg •120ml milk •45g oats •Pinch salt, •1tsp baking powder. ***Blend and pour on a non-stick pan. Serve with a few chopped strawberries***	*Smoked Salmon Bagel* •75g smoked salmon •2 tbsp cream cheese) •Grapefruit
Snack	•Peanut butter on 1 slice wholemeal bread	•1 hard-boiled eggs •1 apple	•1 orange •Handful of almonds	•1 turkey slice •1 cheese slice •1 cracker	•Greek yoghurt	•*Chocolate-peanut butter Smoothie* (page 52)	•1 handful mixed berries •1 handful mixed nuts
Lunch	*Tuna Salad* •1 tin tuna •Baby spinach •Balsamic vinaigrette	*Salmon Salsa* •Small tin salmon •Salsa •3 slices melon •Baby spinach	*Chicken noodles* •Microwave rice noodles •150g cooked chicken breast chunks •Baby spinach •Chopped mushrooms	*Chicken salad* •125g cooked chicken breast •Baby spinach •Walnuts •Cucumbers	*Spicy Tuna Salad* •1 tin tuna •2 tbsp soy sauce •2 tsp wasabi •1 tbsp rice wine vinegar •Mixed greens. •Peppers	*Tuna Melt Sandwich* •1 tin tuna •2 slices wholemeal bread •½ sliced avocado •1 slice cheddar cheese *Grill for 4mins*	*Traditional Roast* •1 roasted chicken breast •1 large potato, quartered and roasted in olive oil •Steamed broccoli, green beans and carrots. •Low-salt Bisto gravy
Snack	•Banana and almonds	•1 hard-boiled egg •1 orange	•60g cottage cheese	•1 turkey slice •1 cheese slice •1 cracker	•1 handful walnuts •1 apple	•Greek yoghurt	•110g ice cream
Dinner	*Steak* •125g Cajun-rubbed sirloin •Griddled onion and courgette •Steamed spinach	*Grilled Chicken* •125g grilled chicken breast, topped with ½ avocado •Grilled asparagus and squash	*Prawn & chicken kebabs* •50g king prawns •125g chicken breast •Onion, quartered •Red and green peppers, chopped *Skewer all the above and grill* •Kale and ½ avocado salad	*Burger* •Grass-fed burger (less than 10 percent fat •Sautéed peppers, onions, and mushrooms	*Chilli* •1 onion, chopped •3 red chillies, chopped and •1 tsp chilli powder •400g lean mince •1 tin kidney beans •2 tins chopped tomatoes ***Brown the onion; fry with the chilli mix; add the rest of the ingredients one by one. Simmer for 20 minutes. Makes 4 portions. Serve with coleslaw.***	*Chilli* •Unless you have a big family there should be at least one portion left over from last night.	*Grilled Salmon* •125g grilled salmon topped with slow-roasted plum tomatoes •Broccoli and lime tender-stem •Spinach and kale salad

ASIAN SALMON BURGERS

Prep 12 mins **Cook** 11 mins **Serves** 4

- 450g skinless salmon fillet, cut into chunks
- 125g fresh wholemeal breadcrumbs
- 1 large egg
- 2 cloves garlic, chopped
- 2 tsp reduced-salt soy sauce
- ½ tsp dark sesame oil
- 2 spring onions, chopped
- 4 tbsp pickled ginger
- 2 tbsp toasted sesame seeds
- 2 handfuls baby spinach

1 In a food processor, blend the salmon, breadcrumbs, egg, garlic, soy sauce, oil, spring onions, and 2 tablespoons of ginger. Pulse until coarsely chopped. Form into 4 equal patties. Top with sesame seeds.

2 Heat a large nonstick pan coated with a little cooking oil over medium heat. Put the burgers sesame-seed side down in the pan. Cook for 5 mins. Flip and cook for 5 minutes longer, or until done.

3 Serve with the spinach and the rest of the ginger.

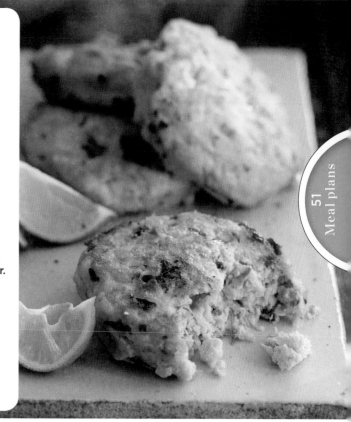

51 Meal plans

BEEF, VEGETABLE, AND ALMOND STIR-FRY

Prep 10 mins **Cook** 15 mins
Serves 4

- 185g rice
- 450g steak, sliced ½cm thick
- 3 tsp reduced-salt soy sauce
- 2 tsp toasted sesame oil
- 1 tbsp grated fresh ginger
- 2 cloves garlic, finely chopped
- 2 medium carrots, thinly sliced
- 1 medium onion, chopped
- 1 red pepper, thinly sliced
- 225g sugarsnap peas
- 3 tbsp sliced almonds
- 2 tbsp hoisin sauce

1 Cook the rice according to the packet directions.

2 Toss the steak with 2 tsp of the soy sauce. Heat 1 tsp of the oil in a large pan over medium-high heat. Add the ginger and garlic. Stir fry for 30 seconds. Add the steak and stir fry for 2-3 mins. Set aside on a plate.

3 Return the pan to the heat, add the rest of the oil, carrots, onion, and pepper. Cook for 3 mins. Stir in the snow peas and almonds. Cook for 2 mins.

4 Add the steak and juices, the hoisin sauce, and 1 tsp soy sauce. Cook for 1 min. Serve over the rice.

SPICED FISH TACOS

Prep 4 mins **Cook** 7 mins
Serves 2

- 150g seabass fillet
- Pinch of salt and black pepper
- Pinch of cumin and chilli powder
- 1 tsp olive oil • 2 corn tortillas
- 3 chopped tomatoes
- 30g finely sliced green cabbage
- 1 tbsp fresh coriander • 1 tsp lime juice

1 Preheat the grill. Season the fish. Grill (or cook in 1 tsp olive oil over medium heat) for 5 mins. Flip and cook for 2 more mins.

2 Divide the fish between the tortillas. Serve with tomato, cabbage, coriander, and lime juice.

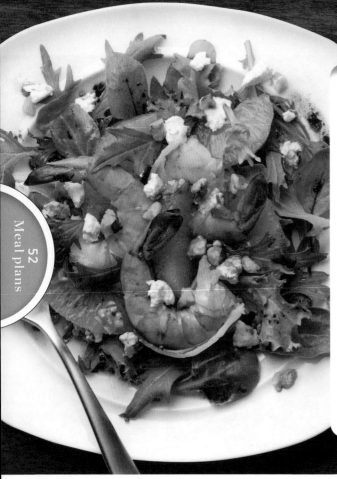

SPECIAL PRAWN SALAD

Prep 10 mins **Serves** 4

- 2¼ tablespoons white wine vinegar
- ½ teaspoon salt
- ½ teaspoon chilli powder
- 3 tablespoons extra-virgin olive oil
- 1 round lettuce, torn into pieces
- 2 grapefruits, cut into segments
- 2 avocados, peeled and sliced
- 275g precooked prawns
- 1 spring onion, including top, thinly sliced
- 4 teaspoons chopped coriander

1 Combine the vinegar, salt, and chilli powder in a small bowl. Whisk in the oil.

2 Put the lettuce on a serving plate or place on 4 individual salad plates. Arrange the grapefruit, avocados, and prawn over the lettuce. Sprinkle with the spring onion and coriander.

3 Drizzle the salad with the chilli dressing.

CHOCOLATE-PEANUT BUTTER SMOOTHIE

Prep 3 mins **Serves** 1

- 1 scoop chocolate protein powder
- 1 tablespoon cacao powder
- 1 tablespoon peanut butter
- 175ml almond milk
- 4 ice cubes

1 In a blender, combine the protein powder, cacao powder, peanut butter, almond milk, milk, and ice cubes. Blend and serve.

BETTER-FOR-YOU EGG SALAD

Prep 15 mins **Cook** 10 mins **Serves** 2

- 4 large eggs
- 225g soft silken tofu
- 4 teaspoons brown mustard
- ½ teaspoon salt
- A few drops hot pepper sauce
- 1 chopped onion
- 15g chopped parsley

1 In a medium saucepan, place the eggs in cold water to cover by several inches. Bring to a boil. Remove from the heat, cover, and let stand for 12 minutes. Run the eggs under cold water until chilled. Peel, halve, and transfer to a large bowl.

2 Add the tofu, mustard, salt, and hot sauce, and mash until some small chunks remain. Fold in the onion and parsley. Cover and chill until serving time.

Week 2

MONDAY

Breakfast
Country Omelette
- 2-egg omelette
- Spinach
- Mushrooms
- Onions
- Peppers
- Feta cheese

Snack
- Greek yoghurt with blueberries and blackberries

Lunch
Chicken Teriyaki
- 125g chicken breasts marinated in 3 tbsp teriyaki sauce and grilled for 20 minutes
- Roasted butternut squash
- *If you are at work you can make this up the night before*

Snack
- Apple
- Handful peanuts

Dinner
Mustard pork chops
- 175g pork chops glazed with Dijon mustard
- Sweet potatoes
- Broccoli

TUESDAY

Breakfast
Mini Fry-Up
- 1 rasher bacon
- 2 fried eggs
- Grapefruit

Snack
Chocolate Peanut Butter Smoothie (page 52)

Lunch
Chicken Fajitas
- 75g chicken breast sliced
- Onion
- Peppers
- 1 jalapeño chilli
- Coriander
- Cumin
- *Fry up the above the night before and refrigerate. Serve in a tortilla wrap*

Snack
- Banana
- Handful peanuts

Dinner
Big Salmon Salad
- 125g salmon seasoned with salt and pepper, and drizzled with olive oil
- Side salad with cucumber, artichoke, broccoli, and tomatoes

WEDNESDAY

Breakfast
Super Cereal
- Cereal of choice with more than 3 grams of fibre,
- 1 sliced banana
- 1 tbsp flaxseed
- 2 hard-boiled eggs

Snack
- ½ melon
- Handful almonds

Lunch
Salmon Salad
- 125g grilled salmon (cooked with last night's salmon)
- Spinach and rocket salad

Snack
- Small pot plain Greek yoghurt

Dinner
Turkey Meatballs
- 125g extra-lean turkey mince
- 1 clove garlic
- ¼ onion
- 4 cream crackers
- 3 tablespoons tomato sauce
- *Chop finely, roll into balls and bake for 30 minutes, along with...*
- Peppers
- Butternut squash

THURSDAY

Breakfast
Porridge Plus
- 30g porridge, cinnamon, ¼ small handful raisins
- 2 low-fat sausages

Snack
- 1 kiwi
- Handful peanuts

Lunch
Tuna Melt Sandwich
- 1 tin tuna
- 2 slices wholemeal bread
- ½ sliced avocado
- 1 slice cheddar cheese
- *Grill if possible*

Snack
- Small pot plain Greek yoghurt

Dinner
Grilled Seafood
- 50g calamari
- 50g prawn
- Chard
- Shallots
- *Cook the lot under the grill or in a griddle pan*

FRIDAY

Breakfast
Breakfast Burrito
- 2 eggs scrambled
- Mozzarella cheese, grated
- Tomato, onions, peppers and avocados, sliced
- Tortilla wrap

Snack
- Apple
- Handful peanuts

Lunch
Greek Chicken Wrap
- 125g cooked chicken breast
- Baby spinach
- Peppers
- Black olives
- Sun-dried tomatoes
- Feta cheese
- 2 tbsp hummus
- Tortilla wrap

Snack
- ½ pint milk

Dinner
Roasted Fish and Veg
- 125g roasted halibut
- Roasted broad beans, yellow squash and shallots

SATURDAY

Breakfast
Protein Berry Smoothie
- 1 scoop vanilla protein powder
- ¼ pint milk
- Strawberries
- Blueberries
- Blackberries
- Handful spinach
- 4 ice cubes
- *Blend and serve*

Snack
- 1 slice cheese
- 1 apple

Lunch
Spicy Beef Stir-fry
- 100g lean steak
- Peppers
- Onions
- Mushrooms
- Sugarsnap peas
- Bean sprouts
- 2 tbsp soy sauce
- Chilli sauce to taste
- *Stir-fry together*

Snack
- 2 hard-boiled eggs

Dinner
Cream Cheese Chicken
- 1 chicken breast
- Cream cheese
- Bacon
- *Slice the chicken fill it with cheese, wrap it in bacon. Roast for 25 mins.*
- Peas and carrots

SUNDAY

Breakfast
Mexican Scrambled Eggs
- 2 eggs,
- Chopped tomatoes, onions, spinach, and peppers
- 30g grated cheese
- 100g salsa

Snack
- Orange
- Handful of almonds

Lunch
Soba Noodle Chicken Pad Thai
- 100g soba noodles,
- 125g chicken
- Peas
- Carrots
- Water chestnuts
- Handful peanuts
- *Stir-fry and add 2 tsp chilli sauce and 2 tsp soy sauce at the end*

Snacks
- 60g cottage cheese
- 2 crackers

Dinner
Steak
- 125g Cajun-rubbed sirloin
- Griddled onion and courgette
- Steamed spinach

MONDAY

Breakfast
Power Protein Porridge
- Porridge oats
- 1 scoop protein
- 1 handful berries
- ¼ pint milk

Snack
- Handful of almonds

Lunch
Sweet Salmon Salad
- 125g cooked salmon (tinned is fine)
- Rocket
- Romaine lettuce
- Cherry tomatoes
- 40g pecans
- 1 satsuma
- Dash olive oil

Snack
- 1 slice cheese
- 1 apple

Dinner
Chicken Stir-Fry
- 175g chicken
- Sugarsnap peas
- Spinach
- Spring onions
- Mushrooms
- Water chestnuts,
- Handful peanuts
- Serve over 75g brown rice

TUESDAY

Breakfast
Spicy Omelette
- 2 eggs
- Spinach
- Mushrooms
- Cheddar cheese
- Salsa

Snack
- 1 slice cheese
- 1 apple

Lunch
Greek Chicken Wrap
- 125g cooked chicken breast
- Baby spinach
- Peppers
- Black olives
- Sun-dried tomatoes
- Feta cheese
- 2 tbsp hummus
- Tortilla wrap

Dinner
Steak and Salad
- 125g grilled sirloin, sliced
- Baby spinach
- Carrots, grated
- Cucumber
- Radish

Snack
Protein Pudding
- 1 tbsp almond butter
- 1 scoop protein powder
- 75ml almond milk
- 1 banana, chopped
Freeze for 1 hour and serve

WEDNESDAY

Breakfast
Strawberry-Banana Protein Smoothie (page 60)

Snack
- 2 handfuls grapes
- 1 slice cheese

Lunch
Chicken & Sweet Potato
- 1 cooked chicken breast
- Sweet potato, microwaved for 6min
- Baby leaf spinach
- Olive oil and Balsamic vinegar dressing

Snack
- 75g ham, sliced
- 2 crackers

Dinner
Chilli
- 1 onion, chopped
- 3 red chillies, chopped and seeded
- 1 tsp chilli powder
- 400g lean mince
- 1 tin kidney beans
- 2 tins chopped tomatoes
Brown the onion, add the rest of the ingredients one by one. Simmer for 20 minutes. Serves 4. Serve with coleslaw.

THURSDAY

Breakfast
Spinach, Mushroom, and Cheese Omelette
- 2 eggs
- 30g cheddar
- Spinach
- Mushrooms

Snack
- 60g cottage cheese
- 2 crackers

Lunch
Tuna Melt Sandwich
- 1 tin tuna
- 2 slices wholemeal bread
- ½ sliced avocado
- 1 slice cheddar cheese
Grill if possible

Snack
- Handful strawberries
- Handful peanuts

Dinner
Chilli
- Unless you have a big family there should be at least one portion left over from last night.

FRIDAY

Breakfast
Berry Good Bacon & Eggs
- 2 scrambled eggs
- 1 rasher bacon
- 1 handful mixed berries

Snack
- 75g beef jerky (or 3 cooked beef slices)
- 2 celery sticks

Lunch
Protein Salad
- 75g cooked chicken slices
- 1 hard-boiled egg
- Romaine lettuce
- Cherry tomatoes,
- Handful sliced almonds,
- 1tsp dressing

Snack
- Apple
- Handful peanuts

Dinner
Lime Chicken
- 125g grilled chicken fried in lime-butter sauce (juice of 2 limes, knob butter)
- Mashed butternut squash
- Steamed spinach and asparagus

SATURDAY

Breakfast
Pineapple-Banana Breeze
- 1 scoop vanilla protein powder
- 175ml almond milk
- 115g pineapple chunks
- 1 banana
- 1 teaspoon vanilla extract
- 4 ice cubes
Blend and serve

Snack
- Peanut butter on wholemeal toast

Lunch
- 1 chicken breast, grilled
- ½ avocado
- Asparagus and courgette

Snack
- 1 slice cheese
- 1 handful of walnuts

Dinner
Grilled Prawn and Scallops
- 50g prawns
- 50g scallops
- 90g cooked quinoa
- Steamed broccoli and carrots

SUNDAY

Breakfast
Yoghurt and Berries
- 245g plain Greek yoghurt
- 1 handful fresh cherries

Snack
- 1 hard-boiled egg
- Apple

Lunch
Burger Salad
- Grass-fed burger
- Blanched kale with butter

Snack
Berry Bliss Smoothie
- 125ml almond
- 125ml water
- 1 scoop vanilla protein powder
- 3 handfuls mixed berries,
- 4 ice cubes
Blend and serve

Dinner
Fish Tacos
- 125g grilled halibut
- 2 corn tortillas
- ¼ sliced avocado
- 2 tbsp salsa,
- Romaine lettuce,
- Mixed peppers
- Red onions, chopped
- ½ sliced jalapeño

GRILLED CHICKEN AND PINEAPPLE SANDWICH

Prep 40 mins **Cook** 12 mins
Serves 4

- 4 boneless, skinless chicken breasts (175g each)
- Teriyaki sauce
- 4 slices emmental cheese
- 4 pineapple slices
- 4 wholemeal rolls or large lettuce leaves for wrapping
- 1 red onion, thinly sliced
- Jalapeño peppers

1 Combine the chicken and teriyaki sauce in a plastic bag. Marinate for at least 30 mins (up to 12hrs max).

2 Preheat the grill. Remove the chicken from the bag and place on the grill. Cook for 4-5 mins on one side. Flip and top each with cheese. Continue cooking until the cheese is melted and the chicken is lightly browned. Set aside.

3 Add the pineapple and rolls to the grill. Cook for 2mins per side, or until rolls are lightly toasted.

4 Top each roll with chicken, onion, jalapeno slices, and pineapple.

EGG AND AVOCADO BREAKFAST SANDWICH

Prep 4 mins **Cook** 4 mins
Serves 1

- 2 large eggs, lightly beaten
- 1 tablespoon mashed avocado
- 1 small bagel, halved and toasted

1 Coat a small nonstick pan with cooking spray and place over medium heat.

2 Add the eggs and cook until set.

3 Spread the avocado on half of the bagel. Top with the eggs and the remaining bagel half.

55
Meal plans

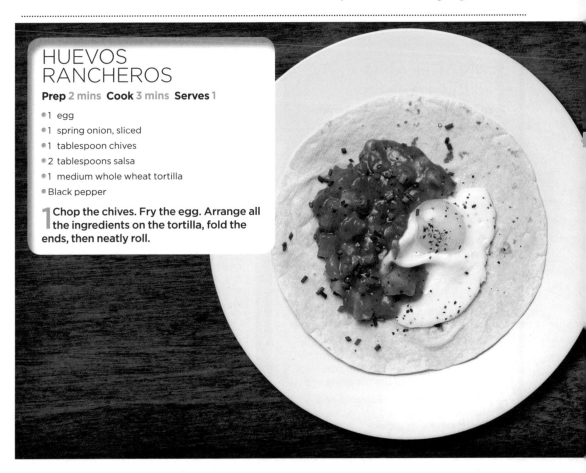

HUEVOS RANCHEROS

Prep 2 mins **Cook** 3 mins **Serves** 1

- 1 egg
- 1 spring onion, sliced
- 1 tablespoon chives
- 2 tablespoons salsa
- 1 medium whole wheat tortilla
- Black pepper

1 Chop the chives. Fry the egg. Arrange all the ingredients on the tortilla, fold the ends, then neatly roll.

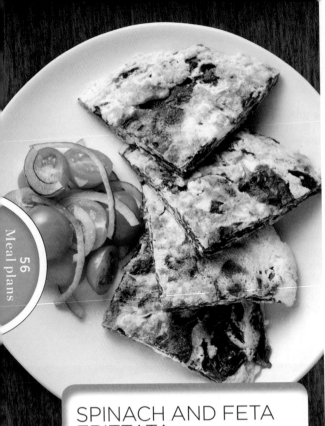

HERBY PORK PITTAS

Prep 45 mins **Cook** 25 mins **Serves** 4

- 2 tbsp olive oil
- 2 tbsp red wine vinegar
- 1 tsp dried oregano
- 4 cloves garlic, crushed
- 550g pork loin, trimmed
- Salt ● Black pepper
- 80g plain Greek yoghurt
- 2 tbsp chopped fresh dill ● 4 wholemeal pittas
- 2 handfuls baby spinach ● 1 tomato, cut in wedges

1 In a resealable bag, blend 1 tablespoon oil, 1 tablespoon vinegar, oregano, and all but a pinch of the garlic. Add the pork, seal the bag, and turn to coat the pork with the marinade. Leave for 30 mins.

2 Preheat the oven to 220°C. Remove the pork from the marinade and discard the marinade. Season the pork, rubbing it with a big pinch salt and grind of black pepper. Heat the remaining tablespoon oil in a large nonstick pan over medium heat. Cook the pork for 5 mins until browned. Transfer to an ovenproof dish and roast in the oven for 15-20 mins, turning once, until the juices run clear. Remove and let rest for 5 mins.

3 In a small bowl mix the yoghurt, dill, the remaining tablespoon vinegar, remaining garlic, and a pinch salt.

4 Thinly slice the pork. Stuff the pitta halves with the pork, spinach,

SPINACH AND FETA FRITTATA

Prep 5 mins **Cook** 15 minutes **Serves** 4

- 3 tablespoons olive oil
- ½ onion, chopped ● 2 cloves garlic, crushed
- 2 big handfuls baby leaf spinach
- 6 large eggs ● 1 slice of bread, in crumbs
- Small handful basil leaves, chopped
- Zest of 1 lemon ● Black pepper ● 120g feta cheese
- Cherry tomatoes ● Red onion

1 In a large pan heat 1 tablespoon of the oil over a medium heat. Add the onion and garlic an cook for 5 minutes. Add the spinach and stir until wilted. Remove from the pan and keep warm.

2 Beat together the eggs, breadcrumbs basil, lemon zest and a grind of pepper.

3 Heat the remaining oil in the pan. Stir the spinach mixture and feta into the egg mixture, then pour into the pan. Heat on low until the top of the frittata is set.

4 Meanwhile half the tomatoes and roughly chop the red onion. Serve with the frittata, cut into slices.

MIXED FRUIT BREAKFAST SMOOTHIE

Prep 2 mins **Serves** 1

- ⅓ pint soy milk
- 20g low-fat ricotta cheese
- 1 scoop vanilla whey protein
- 1 handful frozen cranberries
- 1 handful frozen mixed fruit

1 In a blender or food processor, combine the soy milk, ricotta, whey protein, cranberries and fruit. Whizz for 1 minute, or until puréed and well blended.

Week 4

MONDAY

Breakfast
Smoked Salmon and Scrambled Eggs on Toast (page 59)

Snack
Mixed Fruit Breakfast Smoothie (page 56)

Lunch
Tuna salad
• 1 tin tuna
• Baby spinach
• Balsamic vinaigrette

Snack
• 1 apple
• 2 hard-boiled eggs

Dinner
Asian Salmon Burgers (page 51)

TUESDAY

Breakfast
Huevos Rancheros (page 55)

Snack
• 2 handfuls mixed nuts and raisins

Lunch
Berry Goat Cheese Salad (page 59)

Dinner
Chilli
• 1 onion, chopped
• 3 red chillies, chopped and
1 tsp chilli powder
• 400g lean mince
• 1 tin kidney beans
• 2 tins chopped tomatoes
Brown the onion; fry with the chilli mix; add the rest of the ingredients one by one. Simmer for 20 minutes. Makes 4 portions. Serve with coleslaw.

Snack
• 1 hard-boiled egg
• 1 orange

WEDNESDAY

Breakfast
Strawberry Protein Pancakes
• 1 scoop vanilla protein powder
• 1 egg
• 120ml milk
• 45g oats
• Pinch salt,
• 1tsp baking powder.
Blend and pour on a non-stick pan. Serve with a few chopped strawberries

Snack
• 1 turkey slice
• 1 cheese slice
• 1 cracker

Lunch
Tangy Turkey Ciabatta (page 60)

Snack
Mint Chocolate Chip Smoothie (page 59)

Dinner
Spiced Fish Tacos (page 51)

THURSDAY

Breakfast
Spinach and Feta Frittata (page 56)

Snack
Chocolate Peanut Butter Smoothie (page 52)

Lunch
Spicy tuna salad
• 1 tin tuna
• 2 tbsp soy sauce
• 2 tsp wasabi
• 1 tbsp rice wine vinegar
• Mixed greens.
• Peppers

Snack
• 1 tbsp cottage cheese
• 2 crackers

Dinner
Beef, Vegetable, and Almond Stir-Fry (page 51)

FRIDAY

Breakfast
Mexican Scrambled Eggs
• 2 eggs,
• Chopped tomatoes, onions, spinach, and peppers
• 30g grated cheese
• 100g salsa

Snack
• 1 slice cheese
• 1 apple

Lunch
Grilled Chicken and Pineapple Sandwich (page 55)

Snack
Strawberry-Banana Protein Smoothie (page 60)

Dinner
Grilled salmon
• 125g grilled salmon topped with slow-roasted plum tomatoes
• tender-stem broccoli and lime
• Spinach and kale salad

SATURDAY

Breakfast
Egg and Avocado Breakfast Sandwich (page 55)

Snack
• 1 handful mixed berries
• 1 handful mixed nuts

Lunch
Special Prawn Salad (page 52)

Snack
• 1 apple
• 2 hard-boiled eggs

Dinner
Prawn & chicken kebabs
• 50g king prawns
• 125g chicken breast
• Onion, quartered
• Red and green peppers, chopped
Skewer all the above and grill

SUNDAY

Breakfast
Egg and cheese sandwich
• 2 eggs scrambled
• 1 slice of cheese melted into the eggs
• Toasted English muffin

Snack
• 1 kiwi
• Handful peanuts

Lunch
Better-for-You Egg Salad (page 52)

Snack
• 60g cottage cheese
• 1 handful of almonds

Dinner
Herby Pork Pittas (page 56)

57
Meal plans

Bonus menu 1

MONDAY	TUESDAY	WEDNESDAY	THURSDAY	FRIDAY	SATURDAY	SUNDAY
Breakfast • *Egg and Avocado Breakfast Sandwich* (page 55)	**Breakfast** • *Spinach and Feta Frittata* (page 56)	**Breakfast** *Super Cereal* • Cereal of choice with more than 3 grams of fibre, 1 sliced banana • 1 tbsp flaxseed • 2 hard-boiled eggs	**Breakfast** • *Huevos Rancheros* (page 55)	**Breakfast** • *Smoked Salmon and Scrambled Eggs on Toast* (page 59)	**Breakfast** *Yoghurt and Berries* • 245g plain Greek yoghurt • 1 handful blueberries • 60g granola	**Breakfast** *Mexican Scrambled Eggs* • 2 eggs, • Chopped tomatoes, onions, spinach, and peppers • 30g grated cheese • 100g salsa
Snack • Greek yoghurt with blueberries and blackberries	**Snack** • *Chocolate-peanut butter Smoothie* (page 52)	**Snack** • 2 handfuls mixed nuts and raisins	**Snack** *Berry Bliss Smoothie* • 125ml almond • 125ml water • 1 scoop vanilla protein powder • 3 handfuls mixed berries, • 4 ice cubes *Blend and serve*	**Snack** • 1 slice cheese • 1 apple	**Snack** • Apple and 2 tablespoons peanut butter • ½ pint milk	**Snack** • 1 orange • Handful of almonds
Lunch • *Better-for-You Egg Salad* (page 52)	**Lunch** • *Special Prawn Salad* (page 60)	**Lunch** *Greek Chicken Wrap* • 125g cooked chicken breast • Baby spinach • Peppers • Black olives • Sun-dried tomatoes • Feta cheese • 2 tbsp hummus • Tortilla wrap	**Lunch** • *Berry Goat Cheese Salad* (page 59)	**Lunch** • *Rice Bowls with Prawn and Pak Choi* (page 60)	**Lunch** • *Grilled Chicken and Pineapple Sandwich* (page 55)	**Lunch** *Traditional Roast* • 1 roasted chicken breast • 1 large potato, quartered and roasted in olive oil • Steamed broccoli, green beans and carrots. • Low-salt Bisto gravy
Snack • *Strawberry-Banana Protein Smoothie* (page 60)	**Snack** • ½ melon • Handful almonds	**Snack** • 1 hard-boiled egg • 1 orange	**Snack** • 110g ice cream • 1 handful mixed berries	**Snack** • 3 slices turkey • 1 slice mozzarella cheese • 3 crispbreads	**Snack** • 1 slice cheese • 1 handful of walnuts	**Snack** • 110g ice cream • 1 handful mixed berries
Dinner *Turkey meatballs* • 125g extra-lean turkey mince • 1 clove garlic • 4 cream crackers • ¼ onion • 3 tablespoons tomato sauce *Chop finely, roll into balls and bake for 30 minutes, along with…* • Peppers • Butternut squash	**Dinner** • 1 chicken breast • Cream cheese • Bacon *Slice open the chicken and fill it with cheese, wrap it in bacon then roast for 25 mins* • Peas and carrots	**Dinner** *Steak* • 125g Cajun-rubbed sirloin • Griddled onion and courgette • Steamed spinach	**Dinner** • *Beef, Vegetable, and Almond Stir-Fry* (page 51)	**Dinner** • *Spiced Fish Tacos* (page 51)	**Dinner** *Grilled Prawn and Scallops* • 50g prawns • 50g scallops • 90g cooked quinoa • Steamed broccoli and carrots	**Dinner** • 125g roasted halibut • Roasted broad beans, yellow squash and shallots

SMOKED SALMON AND SCRAMBLED EGGS ON TOAST

Prep 3 mins **Cook** 7 mins **Serves** 1

- 1 slice hearty bread, such as sourdough or wholemeal
- 1 egg
- Salt & pepper
- 25g smoked salmon
- 1 red onion, thinly sliced (optional)
- Capers, fresh dill, 1 lemon (optional)

1 Toast the bread. Meanwhile, in a bowl, whisk the egg with salt and pepper. Pour into a nonstick pan and scramble. Lay the smoked salmon on the toasted bread and top with the scrambled egg. Finish with red onion and capers if you fancy them.

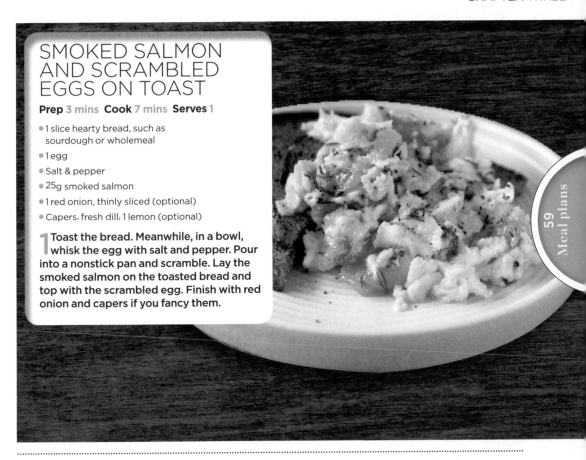

59 Meal plans

BERRY GOAT CHEESE SALAD

Prep 15 mins **Cook** 10 mins **Serves** 1

Dressing
- 1 small handful strawberries
- Juice and zest of ½ orange
- 1½ teaspoons red wine vinegar
- ½ teaspoon sugar
- 2 tbsp fat-free Greek yoghurt
- Pinch salt

1 For the dressing: Combine all the dressing ingredients in a food processor, or whisk together until smooth.

Salad
- 2-3 pecans, crushed
- Big handful baby spinach
- Handful halved strawberries
- 1 handful blueberries
- 1 tomato, cut into eighths
- 2 radishes, thinly sliced
- 1 boneless, skinless chicken breast (175g), grilled
- 1 slice goat cheese

1 For the salad: Toast the pecans in a 200°C oven for 2 mins. Remove from the oven and set aside. In a bowl, mix the spinach, berries, tomato, and radishes. Add the dressing and toss gently.

2 Divide the salad between 2 plates. Place half the chicken on each salad. Top with pecans and goat cheese.

MINT CHOCOLATE CHIP SMOOTHIE

Prep 7 mins **Serves** 1

- 175ml water
- 1 mint tea bag
- 6 ice cubes
- 1 scoop chocolate whey protein powder
- 125g plain Greek yoghurt
- 1 tablespoon cacao powder
- 1 tablespoon cacao nibs or dark chocolate chips

1 Boil the water and let the tea bag steep for 5 to 7 minutes. Discard the bag and pour the tea into a blender with the ice cubes, protein powder, yoghurt, cacao powder and cacao nibs or chocolate chips. Blend and serve.

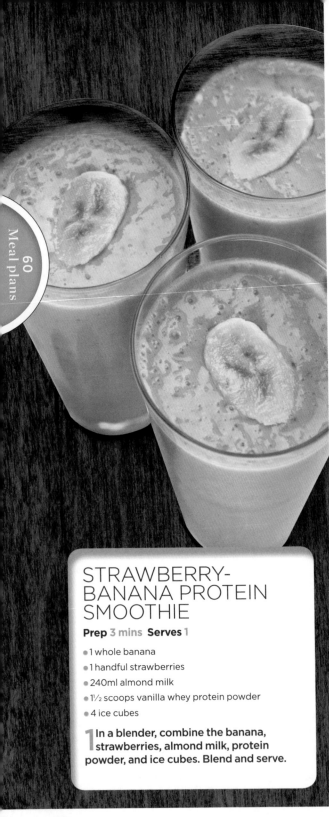

RICE BOWLS WITH PRAWNS AND PAK CHOI

Prep 20 mins **Cook** 10 mins   **Serves** 4

- 1 handful quick-cooking brown rice blend (brown rice, wild rice, basmati and red rice)
- 3 tablespoons ponzu sauce
- 3 tablespoons unseasoned rice vinegar
- 4 teaspoons dark sesame oil
- 2 teaspoons fresh ginger, peeled and grated
- 2 teaspoons brown sugar
- 1 teaspoon hot chilli sauce
- 1 head pak choi, thinly sliced
- 450g cooked prawns
- 2 carrots, grated
- 1 cucumber, peeled, halved lengthwise, seeded, and thinly sliced
- 1 small handful fresh coriander

1 Cook the rice according to packet directions without added salt or fat.

2 In a small bowl, whisk the ponzu sauce, vinegar, 3 teaspoons of the sesame oil, the ginger, brown sugar, and chilli sauce.

3 In a large nonstick pan, heat the remaining sesame oil over medium heat. Add the pak choi and cook 3 to 4 minutes, stirring frequently, or until wilted.

4 Place the rice in 4 bowls. Top with pak choi, shrimp, carrots, and cucumber. Add the dressing and coriander.

STRAWBERRY-BANANA PROTEIN SMOOTHIE

Prep 3 mins **Serves** 1

- 1 whole banana
- 1 handful strawberries
- 240ml almond milk
- 1½ scoops vanilla whey protein powder
- 4 ice cubes

1 In a blender, combine the banana, strawberries, almond milk, protein powder, and ice cubes. Blend and serve.

TANGY TURKEY CIABATTA

Prep 4 mins **Serves** 1

- 1 tablespoon pesto
- 1 ciabatta roll
- 1 handful baby spinach leaves
- 50g turkey slices
- 1 slice mozzarella cheese
- 3 pickle slices

1 Spread the pesto the ciabatta roll. Layer on the spinach leaves, turkey, cheese, and pickle slices.

Bonus menu 2

MONDAY

Breakfast
Breakfast Burrito
- 2 eggs scrambled
- Mozzarella cheese, grated
- Tomato, onions, peppers and avocados, sliced
- Tortilla wrap

Mixed Fruit Breakfast Smoothie (page 56)

Lunch
Tuna Salad
- 1 tin tuna
- Baby spinach
- Balsamic vinaigrette

Snack
- 1 slice cheese
- 1 apple

Dinner
Chicken Stir-Fry
- 175g chicken
- Sugarsnap peas
- Spinach
- Spring onions
- Mushrooms
- Water chestnuts,
- Handful peanuts
- Serve over 75g brown rice

TUESDAY

Breakfast
Power Protein Porridge
- Porridge oats
- 1 scoop protein
- 1 handful berries
- ¼ pint milk

Snack
- 1 slice cheese
- 1 apple

Lunch
Burger Salad
- Grass-fed burger
- Blanched kale with butter

Dinner
Herby Pork Pittas (page 56)

Snack
Protein Pudding
- 1 scoop protein powder
- 75ml almond milk
- 1 tbsp almond butter
- 1 banana, chopped
Freeze for 1 hour and serve

WEDNESDAY

Breakfast
Spicy Omelette
- 2 eggs
- Spinach
- Mushrooms
- Cheddar cheese
- Salsa

Snack
- 2 handfuls grapes
- 1 slice cheese

Lunch
Protein Salad
- 75g cooked chicken slices
- 1 hard-boiled egg
- Romaine lettuce
- Cherry tomatoes,
- Handful sliced almonds,
- 1tsp dressing

Dinner
Steak and Salad
- 125g grilled sirloin, sliced and mixed with...
- Baby spinach
- Carrots, grated
- Cucumber
- Radish

Snacks
Chocolate–Peanut Butter Smoothie (page 52)

THURSDAY

Breakfast
Spinach, mushroom, and cheese omelette
- 2 eggs,
- 1 teaspoon salt,
- 1 teaspoon pepper, 2 tablespoons cheddar cheese, spinach, mushrooms)

Snack
Strawberry-Banana Protein Smoothie (page 60)

Lunch
Sweet Salmon Salad
- 125g cooked salmon (tinned is fine)
- Rocket
- Romaine lettuce
- Cherry tomatoes
- 40g pecans
- 1 satsuma
- Dash olive oil

Snack
- 75g ham, sliced
- 2 crackers

Dinner
Grilled Prawn and Scallops
- 50g prawns
- 50g scallops
- 90g cooked quinoa
- Steamed broccoli and carrots

FRIDAY

Breakfast
Super Cereal
- Cereal of choice with more than 3 grams of fibre,
- 1 sliced banana
- 1 tbsp flaxseed
- 2 hard-boiled eggs

Snack
- 75g beef jerky (or 3 cooked beef slices)
- 2 celery sticks

Lunch
Tuna Melt Sandwich
- 1 tin tuna
- 2 slices wholemeal bread
- ½ sliced avocado
- 1 slice cheddar cheese
Grill if possible

Dinner
Lime Chicken
- 125g grilled chicken fried in lime-butter sauce (juice of 2 limes, knob butter)
- Mashed butternut squash
- Steamed spinach and asparagus

Snacks
Mint Chocolate Chip Smoothie (page 59)

SATURDAY

Breakfast
Strawberry Protein Pancakes
- 1 scoop vanilla protein powder
- 1 egg
- 120ml milk
- 45g oats
- Pinch salt,
- 1tsp baking powder.
Blend and pour on a non-stick pan. Serve with a few chopped strawberries

Lunch
Spicy Tuna Salad
- 1 tin tuna
- 2 tbsp soy sauce
- 2 tsp wasabi
- 1 tbsp rice wine vinegar
- Mixed greens.
- Peppers

Snack
- 1 slice cheese
- 1 handful of walnuts

Dinner
Asian Salmon Burgers (page 51)

SUNDAY

Breakfast
Mixed Fruit Breakfast Smoothie (page 56)

Snack
- Peanut butter on wholemeal toast

Lunch
Sweet Chicken Salad
- 170g grilled chicken
- Rocket
- Baby spinach,
- Walnuts
- Cucumbers
- Mint leaves
- Orange segments

Snack
- 1 kiwi
- 1 cup plain Greek yogurt

Dinner
Fish Tacos
- 125g grilled halibut
- 2 corn tortillas
- ¼ sliced avocado
- 2 tbsp salsa,
- Romaine lettuce,
- Mixed peppers
- Red onions, chopped
- ½ sliced jalapeño

Build a better...
CUPCAKE

Who doesn't love a cupcake? But at 500 calories a pop, the icing's about the only sweet thing. Here's our DIY (and high-street) guide to a guilt-free version

SPONGE

Just one bakery cupcake contains half your daily saturated fat allowance. Try substituting half the butter in your homemade sponge (1) for olive oil and you'll shave 40% off the fat content. Refined white flour is another evil – the blood-sugar kick and crash it causes is the reason you reach for a second cake. "Make flourless cakes using ground almonds and whipped egg whites, or swap white flour for wholemeal spelt flour, which is much easier on your stomach," advises Lily Jones, aka baker Lily Vanilli. Two cupcakes + half the guilt = our kind of maths.

ICING

That pretty buttercream swirl contains a tablespoon of butter and two tablespoons of icing sugar. Lily has a few nifty work-arounds: "Substitute butter for ripe avocado (2). The icing sugar will preserve the fruit so it doesn't go brown, but the fats are all good ones, plus you get a lovely natural colouring." Low-fat cream cheese with a smidge of icing sugar and blitzed-up strawberries (3) or blueberries (4) also works well.

DECORATION

Sure, sprinkles catch your eye, but they're a bad mix of sugar, corn starch and fat. "Desiccated coconut (5), pomegranate seeds (6) and roasted pecans add texture without a sugar high," says Lily. Top with dark chocolate (7) instead of milk chocolate drops, too. It'll satisfy a craving in half the calories.

FLAVOUR

Swap refined sugar for naturally sweet ingredients that will count towards your five a day. Lily says, "Try root vegetables or courgettes (8) in your batter. Carrots (9) and beetroots (10) are naturally sweet and give a great colour. Vegetables add moisture and flavour without extra sugar and fat." Sold.

CASES

Like David Beckham, all tasty things should come in a beautiful package. Our favourite cases are Meri Meri Pansie Cupcake Cases (£3.25 for 48) (11), Jardin Muffin Cases from Lakeland (£2.99 for 24) (12) and Hope and Greenwood Fairy Cake Cases (£6 for 90) (13). There you have your cake, now you can eat it.

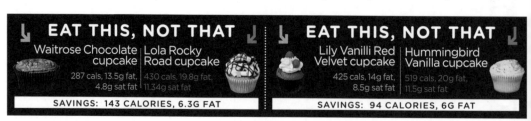

EAT THIS, NOT THAT

Waitrose Chocolate cupcake | Lola Rocky Road cupcake
287 cals, 13.5g fat, 4.8g sat fat | 430 cals, 19.8g fat, 11.34g sat fat

SAVINGS: 143 CALORIES, 6.3G FAT

EAT THIS, NOT THAT

Lily Vanilli Red Velvet cupcake | Hummingbird Vanilla cupcake
425 cals, 14g fat, 8.5g sat fat | 519 cals, 20g fat, 11.5g sat fat

SAVINGS: 94 CALORIES, 6G FAT

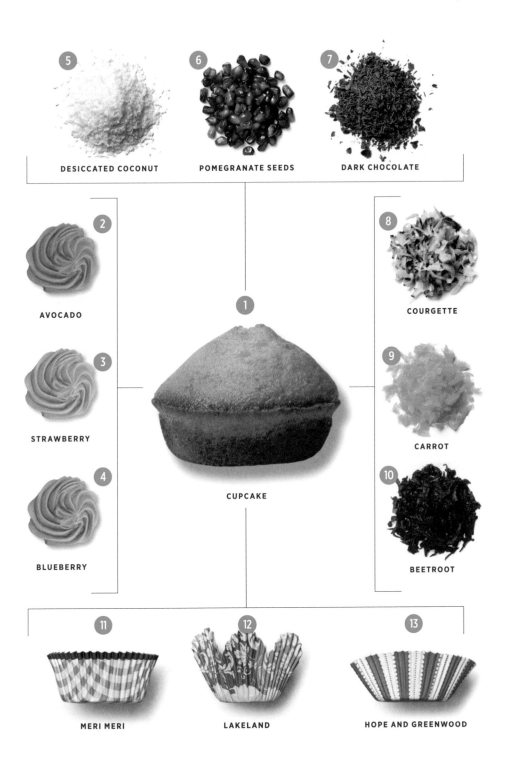

5 DESICCATED COCONUT

6 POMEGRANATE SEEDS

7 DARK CHOCOLATE

2 AVOCADO

3 STRAWBERRY

4 BLUEBERRY

1 CUPCAKE

8 COURGETTE

9 CARROT

10 BEETROOT

11 MERI MERI

12 LAKELAND

13 HOPE AND GREENWOOD

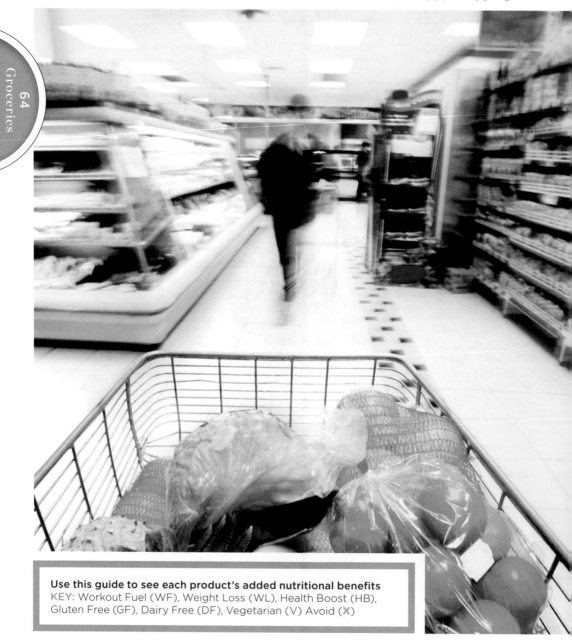

Supermarket sweep

We've scoured the supermarket shelves to find the best (and worst) products for your health and a flat belly. Happy shopping!

Use this guide to see each product's added nutritional benefits
KEY: Workout Fuel (WF), Weight Loss (WL), Health Boost (HB), Gluten Free (GF), Dairy Free (DF), Vegetarian (V) Avoid (✗)

PASTA & GRAINS

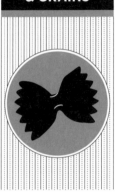

AMOY UDON THICK NOODLES
£1.79, sainsburys.co.uk

(WL)(V)(DF)

It's worth taking note that Sharwood's egg noodles contain 346cal per 100g. These come in at less than half that. Impressive.

Per 100g: 138cal, 1.6g fat

TILDA WHOLEGRAIN BASMATI RICE
£2.49, sainsburys.co.uk

(WF)(GF)(V)

This rice has the bran still intact, giving it a nutty flavour. The calorie content when cooked boils down to only 112cal. One of the lowest around.

Per 100g: 112cal, 0.9g fat

GREAT SCOT QUINOA
£2.18, asda.com

(WL)(V)

A bit like Shaun Ryder, quinoa has an unpleasant coating that needs a good wash. Great Scot's needs no soaking *and* weighs in with healthier stats than any other brand.

Per 100g: 95cal, 2g fat

GAROFALO WHOLE WHEAT FUSILLI
£2.09, ocado.com

(V)(WF)(DF)

These twirls have up to 90% more phytonutrients than 'white' pasta. This brand is also one of the leanest out there as well as being organic.

Per 100g: 334cal, 2g fat

THE FRESH PASTA CO CHEESE RAVIOLI
£3.75, asda.com

A quick dinner? Yes, but it's also an easy way to ingest more fat than a Krispy Kreme and more sat fat than 100ml of Ben & Jerry's Phish Food.

Per 125g: 357cal, 18g fat

DAIRY

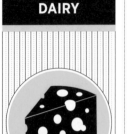

M&S SKIMMED 0.1% FAT MILK **49p, marksandspencer.com**

(WL)(HB)(V)(GF)

All 0.1% milks come in close – Marks' churned out the competition with a lower sat fat content and higher protein count.

Per 100ml: 35cal, 3.4g protein, trace sat fat

SAINSBURY'S 'OMEGA 3' EGGS
£1.65, sainsburys.co.uk

(WL) (HB)(V)(GF)

These eggs have 400mg of EPA and DHA omega-3s, which have been proven to help reduce belly fat. Regular eggs have about 40 mg.

Per egg: 69cal, 4.7g fat

FLORA PRO-ACTIV OLIVE SPREAD
£1.90, waitrose.com

(WL)(HB)(V)(GF)

Lower in cals and sat fat than other 'lighter' spreads like Bertolli, plus 1 tbsp has 2g plant sterols, which impair cholesterol uptake.

Per 10g: 32cal, 0.8g sat fat

CATHEDRAL CITY LIGHTER CHEDDAR
£3, co-operativefood.co.uk

(WL)(V)(GF)

Keeping the protein high and the fat lower than all other cheddars, it also has 120% of your RDA of calcium in 100g.

Per 100g: 311cal, 28.6g protein, 21.8g fat

YEO VALLEY 0% MANGO, PEACH & PASSION FRUIT
£1.40, ocado.com

This yoghurt has 0% fat, but more sugar than a Cornetto. M&S Count On Us Yoghurt has 7.1g sugar.

Per 150g: 119cal, 20.7g sugars, 0g fat

65
Groceries

BREAD & CEREAL

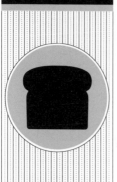

THE FOOD DOCTOR MULTI-SEED & CEREAL PITTAS
£1 for 5, waitrose.com

(WL)(V)
These contain less sugar than some wholemeal pittas (Tesco 2g) and the seed mix is great for energy and omega-3.

Per 70g: 157cal, 1.4g sugar

ALPEN NO ADDED SUGAR MUESLI
£4.29, waitrose.com

(WL)(V)
This only has raisins for sweetness and no added sugar, so it has more than 10g less sugar than Dorset Cereals Organic Muesli (18g). Sweet.

Per 45g: 158cal, 7.3g sugar

FUEL NUT LOADED GRANOLA
£3.28, asda.com

(WF)(V)
This granola not only has more protein than other brands but has half the sat fat of other granolas – Kellogg's has 5g.

Per 50g: 235cal, 9.8g fat, 1.9g sat fat

MORNFLAKE OATBRAN
£1.99, waitrose.com

(WF)(HB)(DF)(V)
Great as porridge or in pancakes, its fibre count helps reduce cholesterol, and you cut 8g of carbs from Quaker oats. Nice.

Per 40g: 146cal, 18.9g carbs

WAITROSE LOVE LIFE BAGELS
£1.49, waitrose.com

(DF)(V)
The New York Bakery Co bagel (42g carbs) has the same carb content as 4 slices of Hovis wholemeal bread. These have 33g.

Per bagel: 175cal, 33g carbs

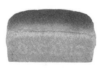

ORGANIC CRUSTY WHOLEMEAL BREAD
£1.30, tesco.com

(WF)(V)
Always look for 100% wholemeal as many brands contain a mix. Buying from the bakery saves about 20cal from a slice of Hovis, too.

Per slice: 66cal, 0.4g fat

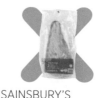

SAINSBURY'S PLAIN NAAN
75p, sainsburys.co.uk

At more than 400cal, one naan bread is the equivalent of eating 8 poppadoms. We know which we'd rather have.

Per serving: 411cal, 14g fat

LARDER

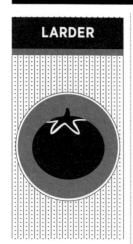

NAPOLINA PEELED PLUM TOMATOES
£1.25, tesco.com

(HB)(DF)(GF)(V)
These are lower in calories than the competition and keep sugars in check. We think they taste the best in spag bol, too.

Per 100g: 23cal, 3.5g sugars, 0.5g fat

SAINSBURY'S NATURALLY SWEET SWEETCORN
55p, sainsburys.co.uk

(WL)(DF)(GF)(V)
You may think corn is universal, but Tesco's version has 80cal, 13.6g carbs and 1.1g of fat.

Per 100g: 61cal, 10.6g carbs, 0.8g fat

WAITROSE ESSENTIAL CANNELLINI BEANS
67p, waitrose.com

(WF)(HB)(DF)(GF)(V)
These high-fibre, large white beans have a firm texture and nutty flavour, and score low on the GI scale.

Per 100g: 89cal, 0.6g fat

MEAT, POULTRY & FISH

DENHAY DRY CURED SMOKED BACON
£3.15, ocado.com

(WF)(DF)(GF)

Cured by hand and slowly matured as well as being a good source of protein. It's also the tastiest around.

Per 100g: 264cal, 20.3g fat

SARTA DE CHORIZO IBERICO RING
£4, sainsburys.co.uk

(WL)(GF)

This is shockingly slender for a Spanish schlong (Tesco's has 39g fat and 465cal per 100g). Perfect if you like it lean.

Per 100g: 278cal, 20.9g fat

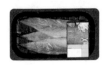

ASDA SMOKED MACKEREL FILLETS
£3, asda.com

(WF)(DF)(GF)

With high levels of omega-3 – beneficial for heart health – this is also one of the cheapest and tastiest.

Per 100g: 295cal, 23.6g fat

THE BLACK FARMER ORGANIC CHICKEN
£6.82, ocado.com

(WF)(DF)(GF)

'Organic' does not automatically denote quality, but these chucks have run free, and have more protein than most.

Per 100g: 148cal, 32g protein, 2.2g fat

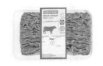

EXTRA LEAN BEEF STEAK MINCE
£4.50, sainsburys.co.uk

(WL)(GF)(DF)

It's a close race between the supermarkets in terms of nutrition (except you, Waitrose – 10g fat) but this one is first over the line.

Per 100g: 123cal, 4.5g fat

DANEPAK HONEY ROAST HAM
£1, sainsburys.co.uk

(WF)(DF)(GF)

If you like your ham sandwiches, this is the pick of the pig as it is lower in all categories than other brands.

Per 100g: 107cal, 19.4g protein, 3g fat

JEAN CABY COCKTAIL SALAMI
£3.49, waitrose.com

Salami is generally bad, but one of Mr Caby's sausages is almost as bad as eating four Snickers' worth of fat.

Per 100g: 516cal, 44g fat

WAITROSE ALBACORE TUNA
£3.20, waitrose.com

(WF)(HB)(DF)(GF)

Always go for tuna in spring water – don't ruin it with fatty oils or brine. This one has a 10cal saving over a tin of John West to boot.

Per 80g: 81cal, 1.1g fat

BAXTER'S HEALTHY MINESTRONE SOUP
£1.14, ocado.com

(HB)(V)

What does this have over its many rivals? Wholemeal pasta. So although other soups have fewer calories this has up to twice the fibre.

Per 100g: 39cal, 0.2g fat

HEINZ BEANZ REDUCED SUGAR AND SALT
53p, asda.com

(DF)(GF)(V)

There is only one brand on top of the beanstalk, and their 'reduced' variety cuts the numbers in all the right places.

Per 100g: 70cal, 0.2g fat

HEINZ SPAGHETTI HOOPS **60p, mysupermarket.com**

Low in cals, great. Low in fat, brilliant. More sugar than a Cadbury's Twirl? Not so great. There's a reason kids love them so much.

Per tin: 212cal, 17g sugar, 1g fat

SNACKS

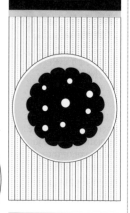

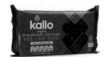

KALLO BELGIAN DARK CHOCOLATE RICE CAKE THINS
£1.59, ocado.com

(WL)(HB)(V)
These have half the sugar and fat and 49cals less per biscuit than a chocolate Hobnob.

Per thin: 30cal, 0.1g sugars, 0.2g fat

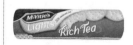

MCVITIE'S LIGHTS RICH TEA BISCUITS
£1.09, tesco.com

(WL)(V)
The Digestive is 70% wholemeal oats, but still contains twice the calories and three times the fat of a Rich Tea. Go figure!

Per biscuit: 36cal, 0.9g fat

TYRRELL'S SWEET & SALTY POPCORN
£1.59, tesco.com

(WL)(HB)(V)(GF)
Butterkist has 11g sugar per 20g, so consider a kernel swap. Tyrrells has far less sugar and keeps carbs and cals in check.

Per 20g: 96cal, 9.8g carbs, 4g sugars, 4.6g fat

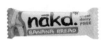

NAKD BANANA BREAD BAR
75p, tesco.com

(WL)(V)(DF)
At under 100cals, this cake-like bar is made from raw fruit, oats and nuts and has fewer calories and carbs than other 'healthy' bars.

Per bar: 92cal, 16g carbs

WALKERS SEA SALTED SUNBITES
£1.79, tesco.com

(WL)(V)
Don't be fooled by some low-cal crisps – most are quick-fried nutritional vacuums. These bags are 67% wholegrain, a third of your RDA.

Per bag: 117cal, 5.4g fat

GREEN & BLACKS 85% DARK CHOCOLATE
£2, tesco.com

(WL)(V)
Watch your percentages – Waitrose Dark Belgian choc is only 48% cocoa, with 11.9g sugar from the rest. G&B's is 85% cocoa – and has 71% less sugar.

Per 25g: 160cal, 3.5g sugar

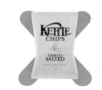

KETTLE CHIPS LIGHTLY SALTED
70p, sainsburys.co.uk

This lard-laden bag carries 12g fat per pack – more than if you chomped down half a Pizza Express Margherita (8.3g).

Per 40g: 205cal, 12g fat

CONDIMENTS

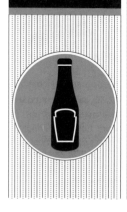

TESCO REDUCED SUGAR & SALT KETCHUP
99p, tesco.com

(WL)(HB)(V)(DF)
At half the sugar content of Heinz Reduced Sugar and Salt ketchup (3g) and fewer calories – there is only one winner.

Per tbsp: 12cal, 1.6g sugar

COLMAN'S WHOLEGRAIN MUSTARD
99p, tesco.com

(WF)(HB)(V)
This has more protein and half the carbs (2.8g) and sugars (1.4g) of Colman's English mustard.

Per tbsp: 23cal, 1.3g carbs, 0.8g sugar, 1.3g protein

VITA D'OR LIGHTER THAN LIGHT MAYONNAISE
99p, lidl.co.uk

(WL)(V)(GF)
We thought that at 11cal per tbsp, Hellmann's Lighter Than Light mayo couldn't be beaten. But this undercuts its rival.

Per 1 tbsp: 10cal, 0.5g fat

INTOLERANCES

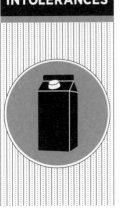

ALPRO ALMOND MILK UNSWEETENED
£1.49, ocado.com

(DF)(GF)(V)

This almond milk is 100% plant based, has half the cals of soya and provides the same amount of calcium as a cup of cow's milk.

Per 100ml: 13cal, 1.1g fat

DOVE'S FARM ORGANIC PASTA
£2, tesco.com

(WF)(DF)(GF)(V)

Cook up your favourite pasta dish minus the wheat, milk, salt, nuts or eggs with the same amount of nutrients as wholemeal pasta.

Per 100g: 338cal, 1.5g fat

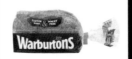

WARBURTON'S GLUTEN & WHEAT-FREE BROWN BREAD
£2.48, asda.com

(WL)(DF)(GF)(V)

Some gluten-free options have added salt to make up for a slight lack of flavour. Warburton's is low in salt, high in flavour.

Per slice: 73cal, 2.2g fat

DOVE'S FARM SPELT FLOUR
£1.99, tesco.com

(DF)(V)

Spelt flour is more easily digested than wheat, due to its higher water solubility. This flour makes baked goods much lower in GI.

Per 100g: 330cal, 2.5g fat

DELAMERE SWEETENED SOYA
£1.30, ocado.com

High in phytic acid, a substance that blocks the body's ability to absorb minerals, soya milk also blocks the hormone oestrogen.

Per 100ml: 39cal, 1g fat

COOKING SAUCES

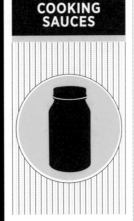

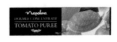

NAPOLINA TOMATO PUREE
99p, tesco.com

(WL)(HB)(V)(GF)(DF)

This contains just one ingredient: tomatoes. It's free from the acidity regulators and sugar found in other brands and is the lowest in calories.

Per tbsp: 11cal, 0.1g fat

THAI TASTE GREEN CURRY PASTE
£1.88, asda.com

(WL)(HB)(V)(GF)

The ingredients for green curry paste are a mix of veg and spices. Red paste has added sugar and modified maize starch. If in doubt, go green.

Per 100g: 106cal, 0.7g fat

DOLMIO LOW-FAT BOLOGNESE SAUCE
£2.08, co-operativefood.co.uk

(WL)(HB)(V)(GF)(DF)

Containing no sat fat and low sugars, this is also one of the tastiest sauces on the shelves.

Per 100g: 28cal, 4.5g sugar, 0.2g fat

SAINSBURY'S LIGHTER GREEN PESTO
£1.50, sainsburys.co.uk

(WL)(HB)

Pesto contains vitamins A and C – important for skin health. Sacla Basil Pesto has 454cal per 100g, this has just 176.

Per 100g: 176cal, 15.3g fat

TASTE THE DIFFERENCE CARBONARA SAUCE
£2.30, sainsburys.co.uk

The 311 cals aren't the worst bit – it's the fact half a pot has almost 70% of your RDA of sat fat.

Per ½ pot: 311cal, 25g fat, 13.8g sat fat

Build a better...
BURGER

Getting a flat belly doesn't have to be incompatible with fast food, particularly if you make it at home. Here's how to scoff a quarter pounder and keep smiling

You want a burger? Us, too. Here's how to build it. Caught on the hop? Oh, alright, we've found the best burger options on the high street, too

BUN
There is 10g sugar in a McDonald's Quarter Pounder with cheese, mostly in the bun. "Go wholemeal (1)," says Sophie Bathgate, founder of Sophie's Steakhouse. "It's low in sugar and salt content." The Food Doctor Multi Seed & Cereal Pitta Bread (2) has 160 calories and tons of fibre. Or go carb-free and use a grilled portobello (3).

CHEESE
We love Cheddar, too, but, at 115 calories and 10g fat per slice, it's no match for feta (4) or Swiss (5) But best is halloumi (6), which has half the fat and 86 calories per chunk. Simmer in water before grilling to reduce salt.

PATTY
The Food Standards Agency says a beefburger must be 62% beef. The rest? 'Mechanically removed meat', fat, rusk, onion powder and dehydrated meat powders. Instead, go DIY. "Use steak mince," says Bathgate. "Most of the fat drains out on the grill." Pat it on a paper towel to further lower fat. Better burgers… no horsing around (7).

ADDED EXTRAS
Iceberg lettuce has minimal taste and, due to its 96% water content, little health benefit. For crunch with nutritional punch, romaine lettuce (8) has 12 times the vitamin A and six times the vitamin C. Tomatoes (9) up your vitamin A, C and E intake while onions (10) have immune-boosting allicin. Salad days.

SAUCE
A burger without ketchup is like Ant without Dec: incomplete. But it has 25% sugar, so freshen up with a salsa (11). "Chop up tomato, avocado and onion to cut through the richness of the meat," says Bathgate. A calorie-free (yes, zero) teaspoon of French mustard (12) peps things up, and a dollop of hummus (13) adds just 27 calories. Saucy.

⬇ EAT THIS, NOT THAT ⬇

The WH burger (above)	McDonald's Big Tasty
516 calories, 8.3g fat, 6g sugar, 1.3g salt	835 calories, 55g fat, 8g sugar, 2.1g salt

SAVINGS: 319 CALORIES, 46.7g FAT

⬇ EAT THIS, NOT THAT ⬇

Subway Veggie Patty	BK Bean Burger
389 calories, 9g fat, 9g sugar, 1.8g salt	590 calories, 20g fat, 13g sugar, 3.8g salt

SAVINGS: 201 CALORIES, 11g FAT

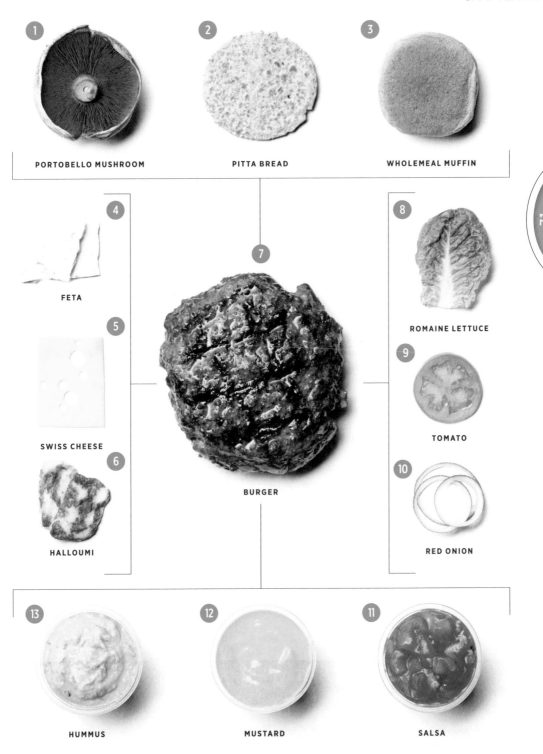

1 PORTOBELLO MUSHROOM

2 PITTA BREAD

3 WHOLEMEAL MUFFIN

4 FETA

5 SWISS CHEESE

6 HALLOUMI

7 BURGER

8 ROMAINE LETTUCE

9 TOMATO

10 RED ONION

11 SALSA

12 MUSTARD

13 HUMMUS

71
Burgers

The protein fix

Upping your daily dose of protein cuts your risk of heart disease, lowers blood pressure and torches fat. Just what the doctor ordered

You'd think if the low-carb craze has taught us anything, it's the importance of protein. According to government guidelines, about 15% of your daily calories should come from the P-stuff. But a study at John Hopkins University in Maryland found upping that to 25% can not only help you lose weight, but also significantly reduce your blood pressure, cholesterol levels and risk of heart disease, too. (So that's another reason to give in to the cheese board then.)

Of course, while that's all very impressive, it doesn't tell you where to get your protein, how much you need or when to eat it. That's where we come in...

PROTEIN IN ACTION
First, a quick biology lesson. Your muscles consist of fibres made of protein. These fibres break down every time you move, so your clever body replenishes them with protein in your food. Eating protein tones your muscles, plus it boosts your metabolism too, since lean muscle burns calories faster than fat. And that isn't the only benefit...

EAT UP, SLIM DOWN
"Many women perceive foods that are rich in protein as being high in calories or fattening," says nutritionist Laura Kruskall, author of the *Fitness Professionals' Guide to Sports Nutrition and Weight Management*. Sure, most proteins will cost you a few more calories than fruit and vegetables, but they are also harder for your body to digest, which means you burn more calories processing them. And what's more, they take longer to leave your stomach, so you feel fuller for longer. In fact, in a study published in *Nutrition Metabolism*, people who increased their protein intake to 30% of their diet ate almost 450 calories fewer a day, losing an average of 11lb in three months. So that's your figure sorted then.

Q I WANT TO TONE UP, BUT IF I INCREASE MY WEIGHTS AND PROTEIN INTAKE HOW DO I AVOID BULKING OUT?

A There are many myths surrounding high protein consumption and weight-training, but neither will leave you looking like a bodybuilder unless you take an extreme approach, says MacDonald. People like the newly buff Jodie Marsh do hours of heavy weight reps every day and follow a strict diet with almost no carbs to drastically reduce their body fat and build (freakily) big muscles.

You'll only bulk out if you keep eating about 200 calories above your daily burn. To tone up, stick to around 1,900 calories and train three to five times per week. This way, you'll lose enough body fat and gain enough muscle to get the definition you want. Download the free MyFitnessPal app to calculate your dietary needs and log the calories and nutrients, including protein, in everything you eat. That should be a weight off your mind.

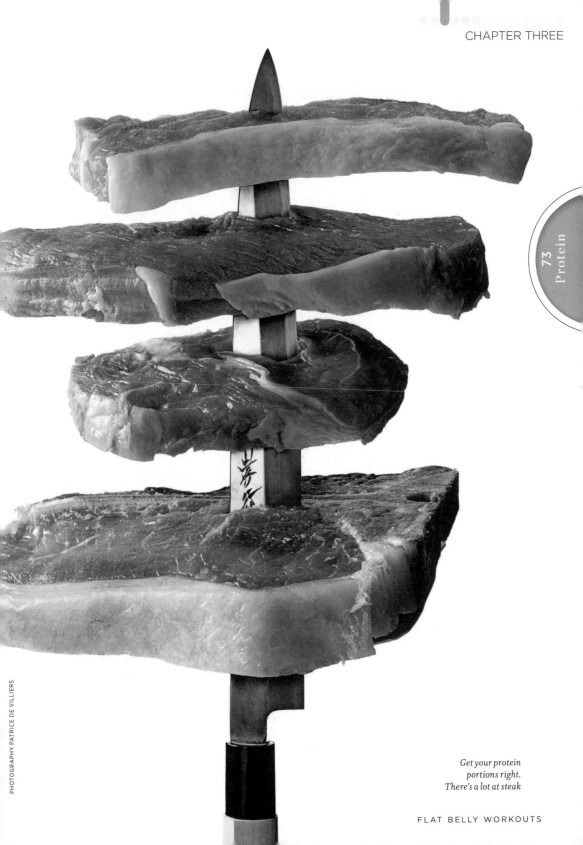

PHOTOGRAPHY PATRICE DE VILLIERS

*Get your protein
portions right.
There's a lot at steak*

FLAT BELLY WORKOUTS

Q ARE ALL PROTEIN SHAKES CREATED EQUAL? I'M A BIT CONFUSED BY THE VARIETY AVAILABLE...

A In a nutshell: no and it depends on your goals. The key ingredient in protein shakes is usually soy, casein powder or whey, a commonly used water-soluble milk protein. Like the other two, it's a complete protein, offering all nine of the amino acids you need, but whey is easiest to digest.

Whichever you pick, avoid any shake powders with less than 75-80g of protein per 100g. Unlike standard powders, 'mass gainer' types have a higher ratio of carbohydrates and fats. And think twice about using soy-based powders, says nutritional scientist Martin MacDonald. "High intakes of soy can affect hormone status and your thyroid," he says. Look for a powder that lists whey protein concentrate or whey protein isolate as the top ingredients.

Studies show having your shake before exercising boosts your metabolic rate compared to if you just eat carbs. So if your aim is to slim, drink it pre-workout. Protein powders can also be added to foods, so get creative.

NAMING SOURCES

Which brings us to our next point – where to get your protein. The first thing you need to know: not all proteins are created equal, says Kruskall. While nuts, whole grains and vegetables such as soy and chickpeas are good sources, they don't contain all nine of the amino acids your body needs to build lean muscle. Your best flat-belly bets are typically found in animal products, including skinless chicken or turkey, seafood, low-fat dairy, eggs, pork tenderloin and lean beef (for a full list, go to nowmuchprotein.com/foods/).

actually too low. Many now recommend eating between 0.8g and 1.1g per pound of your body weight. For a 10-stone woman, that's 112-154g a day – the equivalent of 600g of chicken breast or 1kg of cottage cheese. Yikes. Go for the high end if you're very active – say, running or lifting weights nearly every day – and the low end if you're trying to shift a bit of weight.

You should aim to eat at least 30g of your target at breakfast,

> ## Don't bother exceeding 30g of protein: our muscles cannot use more than that in one go

Another bonus is that all these sources have just two to six grams of fat per 100-calorie serving. If you're a vegan, opt for complete proteins such as tofu, hemp seed or buckwheat.

WEIGH TO GO

Of course, you need to think quantity as well as quality. A growing number of nutritionists believe the current GDAs for protein are

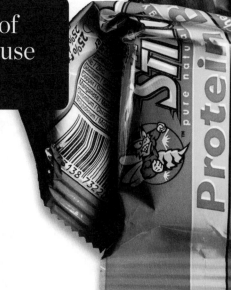

says Donald Layman, professor of nutrition at the University of Illinois. Your body will start drawing on muscle tissue for fuel after fasting all night if you don't replenish your protein stores first thing. Studies show it will also help to regulate your appetite for the rest of the day. Try two eggs and a small pot of low-fat Greek yoghurt (try Danone Oykos, £2.19 for four 110g pots, Waitrose).

Don't bother exceeding your 30g, though. Our muscles cannot use more than that when eaten in one go, adds Suzane Leser, chair of the European Specialist Sports Nutrition Alliance. So spread your intake across your meals. Try snacking on 25g of roasted soy nuts or a boiled egg. Or, if you're dashing from the gym to the office, protein shakes and bars can keep you fuelled up (see our shakes guide below). Which leaves you ready to dazzle like the protein pro you now are.

Q I OFTEN EAT ON THE MOVE. ARE PROTEIN BARS A HEALTHY OPTION?

A Protein bars can be a way to fuel up fast, but make sure you read the labels. Many so-called nutrition bars have partially hydrogenated oils and excess fat and sugar, warns MacDonald. Choose a bar with at least six grams of protein. Try MyProtein High Pro (£1.99), with 29g. If you work out, you'll also need up to 35g of carbs for quick energy, plus up to eight grams of heart-healthy unsaturated fats and six grams of fibre to fill you up. So go ahead and tuck in.

75 Protein

SHAKE UP YOUR FITNESS GOALS

Whether you're looking to tone up, slim down or trim your tum, these four targeted protein shakes provide the winning mix you need to succeed

FAT BURNER

TRY: Blend 30g of a protein blend powder (try Maxitone Sculptress Diet, £24.99 for 700g) with 2tbsp flaxseed powder (£5.66 for 450g) and 400ml of water.

WHY: Flaxseed is very rich in omega-3 fats, which assist in fat loss, as well as lignan antioxidants, which are essential for boosting energy and aiding recovery, especially if you are in the habit of doing plenty of cardio work.

WHEN: Drink this in-between meals or use it to replace a meal heavy in carbs.

TUMMY TRIM

TRY: Whizz up 30g of protein blend (try Body Complete, £60 for 640g), with 1tbsp flaxseed oil (£10.65 for 473ml), 2tbsp oats and 50g strawberries, plus 300ml of water or milk.

WHY: Flaxseed oil is a good source of flab-busting omega-3 fats, while the addition of the oats provides low-GI carbs plus fibre that will help to fill you up.

WHEN: Use this Tummy Trim shake either to replace a snack or as a light meal.

PRE-GYM PUNCH

TRY: Blend 30g of whey protein (try The Good Whey Premium Triple Filtered Protein, 500g, £15.95) with 1 banana, 50g blueberries and 400ml of water.

WHY: Blueberries are full of potassium, which boosts energy, antioxidants and natural sugars, and are packed with a hefty dose of vitamins, too.

WHEN: Drink a third of this shake 20 minutes before your workout, a third during the exercise session and the rest of it afterwards.

MEAL REPLACER

TRY: Mix 30g of protein blend (Herbalife Formula 1 Healthy Meal, £27.60 for 550g), with 1tsp almond butter, 2tbsp yoghurt, 1tsp Barley Grass Powder (try Naturya Organic, £7.99 for 200g) and 2tsp flaxseed powder. Then mix with 400ml of water.

WHY: 'Real meals' are still best for nutrients, so use as many natural foods as you can in your more convenient shake to maximise your intake.

WHEN: In place of a heavy evening meal.

Booze control

Giving up the things you love will make a flat belly unsustainable. So learn to drink smart and you can party when you like and stay trim and hangover free

We're sure you love a good party – but odds are you body is less keen. Sure, you may feel great after that third glass of wine (for a while, at least), but your system is working overtime trying to deal with all those toxins and extra calories. And come the next morning, no one is happy.

Of course, you're still going to drink anyway. But with our smart boozing tactics, you can indulge whilst boosting your immune system, slashing calories and minimising hangovers. Plus, have that post-bender greasy-spoon breakfast you crave – without the guilt.

"Alcohol tolerance is affected by lots of factors," says GP Keith Hopcroft. The basic ones – how quickly you drink, your weight and whether your stomach is full – are well documented. "But odd as it seems, how 'watery' you are also plays a part," says Hopcroft. "Men are 66% fluid, so the booze is diluted out, while women only score 55%, so they tend to get legless more quickly."

There's not much you can do about that, but you can avoid drinks which pack high levels of congeners, by-products of alcohol fermentation that ramp up your hangover. Red wine and darker spirits such as whiskey and tequila contain more of these toxins than white wine and clear spirits such as vodka and gin. In a study, 33% of testers who drank an amount of bourbon relative to their body weight got a severe hangover, compared to just 3% of those who drank vodka. These chemical nasties are the reason your mum told you never to mix your drinks, too. Beer, wine and spirits contain different types of congeners, so when you combine them your body has to work harder to combat all those impurities.

Drinking booze with bubbles makes things even worse. A study at Manchester University found carbonated mixers and drinks such as Champagne get you drunk faster, as the gas helps push the alcohol through your gut into your bloodstream.

So that explains why some drinks hit you harder than others. Now strike back with our scientifically-approved drink swaps and tips to hammer all types of hangover. Headache, what headache?

Women get drunker as our bodies contain less liquids to dilute alcohol than men

NEAR-DEATH HANGOVER

You know this old friend – you wake up and feel like you may die. After vomiting for the third time, you wish you had

The culprits Red wine, dark rum, port.

Sobering facts Diet mixers get you more sloshed, more quickly, than sugary varieties. An Australian study found booze with diet drinks hit testers' bloodstreams 15 minutes sooner and caused 50% higher blood alcohol levels. Sugar takes longer to move through your stomach, slowing alcohol too.

Greasy-spoon cure A bacon butty can help. "Bacon contains amino acids that top up depleted neurotransmitters," says Elin Roberts, of Newcastle University's Centre for Life. Plus, carbs in the bread provide an energy boost. Result!

DRINK THIS, NOT THAT

Avoid a hangover altogether by sticking to one or two and keep your belly flat with these swaps

DRINK THIS	NOT THAT	SAVE
BARCARDI BREEZER ORANGE (275ml) 100cals, 1.1 units	**WKD BLUE** (275ml) 185 cals, 1.4 units	**85** CALORIES
DRY RED WINE (125ml) 100 calories, 1.5 units	**MULLED WINE** (125ml) 253 calories, 1.6 units	**153** CALORIES
BAILEY'S (37.5ml) 117 calories, 1.1 units	**EGGNOG** (250ml) 345 calories, 1.5 units	**228** CALORIES
GIN RICKEY 65 calories, 1 unit	**GIN AND TONIC** 171 calories, 1 unit	**106** CALORIES
MALIBU AND PINEAPPLE 111 calories, 1 unit	**PINA COLADA** 526 calories, 2 units	**415** CALORIES
CORONA LIGHT BEER (330ml) 109 calories, 1.5 units	**LEFFE BLONDE BEER** (330ml) 200 calories, 3 units	**91** CALORIES
VODKA AND SODA 100 cals, 1 unit	**MOSCOW MULE** 185 calories, 2 units	**85** CALORIES

BY MAKING JUST THREE OF THESE SWAPS A WEEK, SAVING A TOTAL AVERAGE OF 500 CALORIES, YOU CAN LOSE AN EXTRA 7LB A YEAR.

Total Save 1,163 cals*

HUNGER HANGOVER

You've got a worse case of the munchies than Cookie Monster and no amount of sugary junk will satisfy it

The culprits Alcopops, sugary cocktails.

Sobering facts Drinking plays havoc with blood sugar, says Dr Thomas Stuttaford, author of *To Your Good Health*. It crashes. Result: raging hunger.

Greasy-spoon cure 1 poached egg, half tin beans, 2 rashers lean bacon, a tomato and 100g mushrooms gives 32g protein for just 400kcal. "This is three of your five-a-day and the protein boosts satiety," says dietician Dr Carrie Ruxton, from the Meat Advisory Panel. Sorted.

DELAYED HANGOVER

Think you've dodged the bullet? Sadly, it's just a small step from still tipsy to sick as a dog – as you'll soon realise

The culprits Strong wines, cocktails.

Sobering facts It takes an hour for your body to process a unit of alcohol. But women have lower levels of the enzyme that breaks it down. Plus, taking oestrogen-added medication like the Pill slows your ability to process alcohol.

Greasy-spoon cure Dr Travis Stork, author of *The Lean Belly Prescription*, suggests a 1-egg omelette with 28g of low-fat cheese and steamed asparagus. "It provides vitamin B12, for energy and amino acids to mop up toxins."

DEPRESSION HANGOVER

Your mood is even lower than your energy levels (and that's before you remember the messy clinch with your boss)

The culprits Er, all alcohol.

Sobering facts The reality is ANY alcohol is a central nervous system depressant. It slows the parts of your brain that control emotions, so you experience exaggerated highs and of course, lows.

Greasy-spoon cure Try nutritional scientist Martin MacDonald's feel-good pancakes. Use 1 egg, 30g of whey protein, a pinch of baking powder and 50g of oats soaked in water. The oats boost mood-regulating serotonin, while the protein prevents depressing blood-sugar slumps.

77 Alcohol

PART
TWO

THE BEST FLAT BELLY EXERCISES

Your ultimate hot-body guide

The following pages are your quick-reference, flat-belly exercise catalogue: 151 moves that work every part of your body and burn fat to reveal your abs

Back when you first started exercising, you probably had a workout that seemed like it provided all the right ingredients you needed to lose weight, fit into your skinny jeans and have more energy. A few reps here, a couple sets there, and you were done. But while your muscles felt like they were working, and sweat dripped from your brow and covered your shirt, the movements you did rarely took off the pounds or came close to creating a slimmer new you.

So what did you do wrong? Technically, nothing. You did the exercises and worked hard. That should be enough to lose weight – but it's not. The secret to a lean body isn't wrapped in just any random mix of exercise. You need variety, but that doesn't mean simply trying every machine in the gym. If you want a flat belly, the movements you perform must challenge your entire body and not just individual muscles like your abs and obliques. When that's achieved, you activate more muscle fibres, burn more calories, and – poof! – start to see your abs.

In order to put an end to your frustrating workouts, we had some of the best fitness minds handpick their favourite exercises. Some exercises may look familiar, like press-ups, squats and lunges. These are part of any great routine. But where most workouts stop is where these workouts actually begin. Our experts created a list of hundreds of moves that will work every muscle in your body, including your abs. We call these the best flat belly exercises ever created because they work you harder and faster for guaranteed results.

As you look through these exercises, it's important that you keep an open mind. You see, some exercises might seem easy and others bizarre. But we promise that these moves will bring out the best in your body and work your body in the ways it needs. Just don't be surprised if you don't see familiar machine-related exercises to tone your legs. Or a whole range of curls to sculpt your arms. If you do what you've always done, you'll get

> If you want a flat belly, the movements you perform must challenge your entire body

the same results you've always achieved. And that's the last thing that we – or our expert fitness advisors – want you to experience.

Not only will these exercises keep you from straying from your workout, they'll actually have you looking forward to your next gym day. And while a great workout doesn't require much equipment, these exercises will provide enough variety that you can do them in your own home or with the expensive kit you'll find at your local training facility. The big difference: these moves are so original that you'll be excited by the challenge of

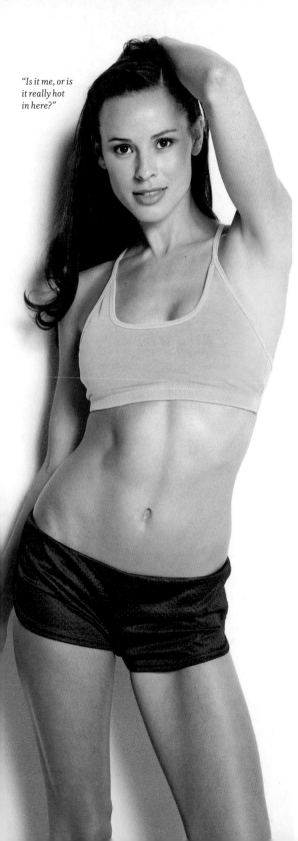

"Is it me, or is it really hot in here?"

something new. And they'll work all of the regions in your core: abs, obliques, transverse abdominis and lower back. Even if you've never lifted a weight before, you'll find that these exercises are more fun than you'd have imagined. But even better – they'll do more than make you sweat. They'll actually produce changes you can see and appreciate.

The best part? These exercises will literally reinvent how you view your belly. You see, there's more than 100 abs exercises in this programme that don't include even the slightest crunching movement – and yet these moves work the muscles in your midsection harder than ever before. What's more, because these exercises simulate real-life movements, you'll build a body that won't experience as many aches and pains. Therein is the beauty of these moves: you'll be working every muscle in your body, sweating, melting calories and transforming your body into a new slim and trim version without even realising it. And in no time, you'll have reshaped your abs, bum, thighs and arms and traded in the older version of you for the gorgeous body you've always wanted.

HOW TO USE THESE EXERCISES

The best way to start familiarising yourself with the exercises in this book is to use one of the tailor-made workouts in Part Three. Simply pick the one that best suits your body aims and use the chart to record exactly how you do with each set. Keeping a record like this will really bolster your motivation. Alongside each move you'll find a page reference so you can flick back to this part and remind yourself exactly how it's done.

Once you've done a few of the workouts in Part Three there's nothing to stop you using the moves in this part to create your own flat belly plan. Just remember that the best workouts include exercises that challenge every muscle in your body – this way you maximise fat-burning, which is the secret of a flat belly. You can use the blank chart on page 222 to create your own routine and record your results. Keeping track of exactly how far you've come is a powerful motivator.

81
The moves

Chapter Four

Chest moves

SCULPT AND TONE YOUR
UPPER BODY WITH THE
BEST EXERCISES

Press-Up

START

Get on all fours, and place your hands on the floor slightly wider than and in line with your shoulders. Your body should form a straight line from your ankles to your shoulders. Squeeze your abs as tight as possible and keep them contracted for the entire exercise.

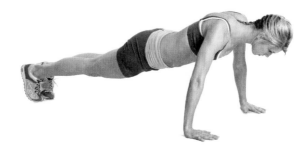

FINISH

Lower your body until your chest nearly touches the floor, making sure that you tuck your elbows close to the sides of your torso. Pause, then push yourself back to the starting position.

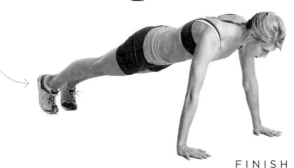

83 Chest

Press-Up Jack

START

Begin in the standard press-up position. Your body should form a straight line from your ankles down to your shoulders.

FINISH

As you lower your body to the floor, jump your feet outward so that they end up shoulder-width apart. As you press your body back up, jump your legs back together and return to the starting position.

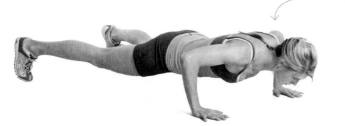

Press-Up Plus

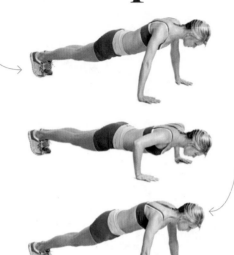

START

Get on all fours and place your hands on the floor slightly wider than and in line with your shoulders. Your body should form a straight line from your ankles to your shoulders. Squeeze your abs as tight as possible and keep them contracted for the entire exercise.

FINISH

Lower your body until your chest nearly touches the floor. Pause, then push yourself back to the starting position. Once your arms are straight, push your upper back toward the ceiling. It's a subtle move, but it should feel like your shoulder blades are flaring out. Pause, then repeat the entire movement.

84
Chest

Pike Press-Up

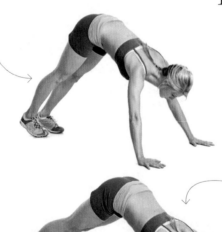

START

Start in a traditional press-up position, then walk your feet towards your hands and raise your hips into the air. Your body should look like an inverted V.

FINISH

Keeping your hips raised, lower your body until your chin nearly touches the floor. Pause, then press back up to the starting position.

T Press-Up

START

Place a pair of dumbbells (preferably hex dumbbells) on the floor about shoulder-width apart. Start in a press-up position and grab the dumbbells. Perform a press-up while holding the dumbbells.

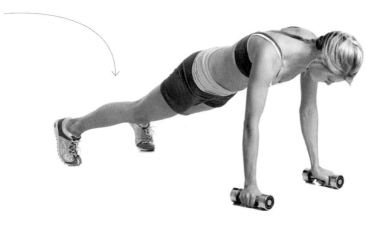

85
Chest

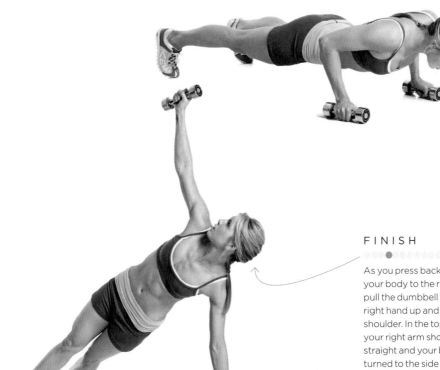

FINISH

As you press back up, rotate your body to the right and pull the dumbbell in your right hand up and above your shoulder. In the top position, your right arm should be straight and your body turned to the side so that you form the letter T. Lower the dumbbell back to the starting position and perform another press-up, and repeat, this time turning to the left.

Press-Up And Step Out

START

Begin in the standard press-up position. Perform a press-up and then "walk" your hands forwards so your body is extended.

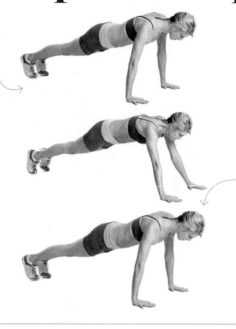

FINISH

Walk your feet forwards so your hands are underneath once again.

Single-Leg Press-Up

START

Begin in the standard press-up position with your body forming a straight line from your ankles to your shoulders. Raise one foot off the floor.

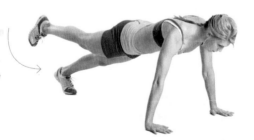

FINISH

Lower your body towards the floor and then press back up, all the while keeping your leg off the floor. Try to perform all reps without lowering your leg.

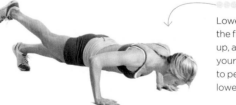

Press-Up With Hand Raise

START

Begin in the standard press-up position with your body forming a straight line from your ankles to your shoulders. Lower your body to the floor and then press back up.

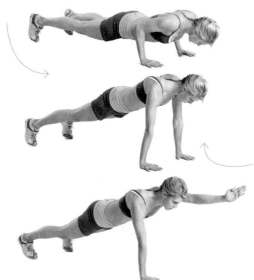

FINISH

As you return to the starting position, raise your right hand so it's in line with your body. Hold for 2 seconds, and then return your hand to the starting position. Do another press-up and then repeat, this time raising your left hand.

87
Chest

Shoulder Touch Press-Up

START

Begin in the standard press-up position with your body forming a straight line from your ankles to your shoulders. Raise one foot off the floor and perform a press-up. As you press back up, take your left hand and touch your right shoulder.

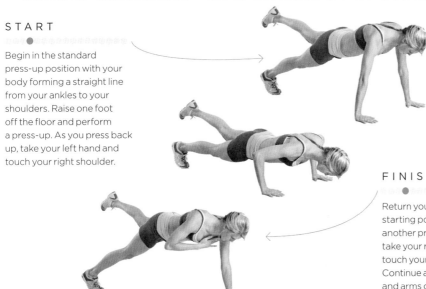

FINISH

Return your hand to the starting position and perform another press-up. This time, take your right hand and touch your left shoulder. Continue alternating legs and arms on each rep.

Incline Press-Up

START

Begin in the standard press-up position, but place your hands on a bench (or a box) instead of the floor. Your body should still form a straight line from your shoulders to your ankles.

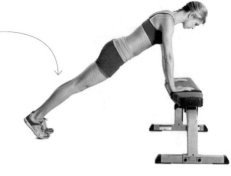

FINISH

Lower your chest to the bench, pause, and then press back up to and return to the starting position.

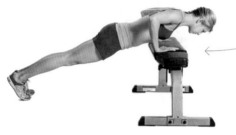

Press-Up Row

START

Place a pair of dumbbells about shoulder-width apart on the floor. Grab the dumbbell handles and position yourself in a press-up position. Lower your body to the floor and then press back up.

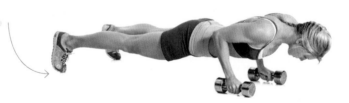

FINISH

Once you're back in the starting position, pull the dumbbell in your right hand up towards the side of your chest. Pause, then return it to the floor and repeat with your left hand. That's 1 rep. Try to prevent your torso from rotating each time you row the weight.

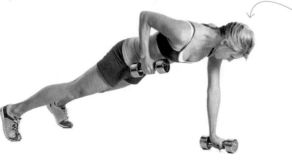

Spider-Woman Press-Up

START

Begin this exercise in the standard press-up position with your body forming a straight line from your ankles to your shoulders.

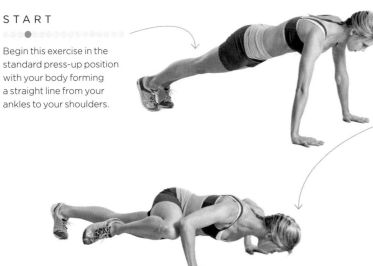

FINISH

As you lower your body towards the floor, lift your right foot up. Bring your right leg out to the side and try to touch your knee to your right elbow. Reverse the movement, then push back up to the starting position. Perform another press-up, but try to touch your left knee to your left elbow. Alternate sides on each repetition.

89
Chest

Alternating Cable Press

START

Attach a D-handle to a cable station and adjust the pulley so the handle is at chest height. With your right hand, grab the high pulley handle and face away from the weight stack. Stagger your feet and make sure the handle is positioned in front of your shoulder. Your arm should be parallel to the floor.

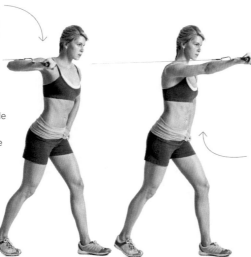

FINISH

Push the handle forward and straighten your arm in front of you. Pause and return to the starting position. Perform all reps on one side, then switch hands and repeat.

Forward Punch

START

Attach a resistance band to a stable object at chest height. With your right hand, grab the band and face away from the anchor point. Stagger your feet and make sure the handle is positioned in front of your shoulder. Your arm should be parallel to the floor.

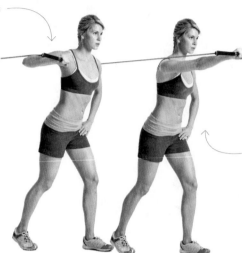

FINISH

Push the band forward and straighten your arm in front of you. Pause and return to the starting position. Perform all reps on one side, then switch arms and repeat.

Swiss Ball Chest Press

START

Grab a pair of dumbbells and lie on your back on a Swiss ball. Raise your hips so that your body forms a straight line from your knees to your shoulders. Your arms should be straight and above your chest, with your palms facing your feet.

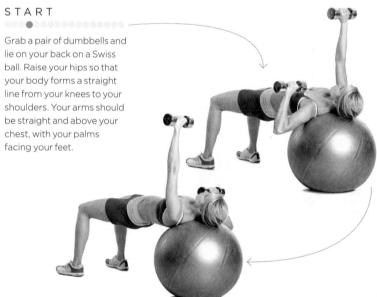

FINISH

Without changing the angle of your hands, lower one dumbbell to the side of your chest. Press it back up to the starting position, then repeat with your other arm. Continue alternating arms until you complete all reps.

Chest Press

START

Grab a pair of dumbbells and lie face-up on a flat bench. Hold the dumbbells above your chest with your arms straight. The dumbbells should be nearly touching, and your palms should be facing your feet.

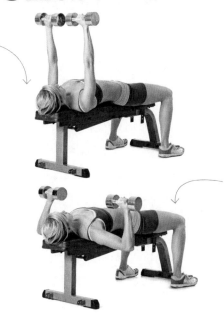

FINISH

Keeping your elbows tucked close to your body, lower the weights to the sides of your chest. Pause, then press the dumbbells back up above your chest.

91 Chest

Incline Press

START

Set an adjustable bench to an incline of 30 to 45 degrees. Grab a pair of dumbbells and lie face-up on the bench. Hold the dumbbells directly above your shoulders with your arms straight.

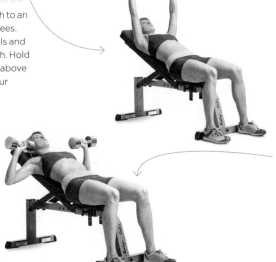

FINISH

Lower the dumbbells to the sides of your chest, pause, and then press the weights back above your chest.

Chapter Five

Back moves

LOOK STUNNING IN ANY
BACKLESS DRESS AND
BALANCE YOUR BODY

Barbell Row

START

Grab a barbell with an overhand grip with your hands about shoulder-width apart. Hold the bar at arm's length, and then bend at your hips and lower your torso until it's almost parallel to the floor. Your knees should be slightly bent and your lower back naturally arched.

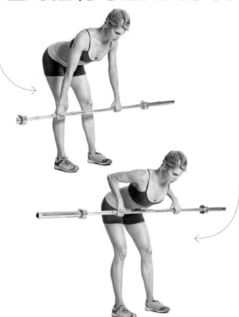

FINISH

Squeeze your shoulder blades together and pull the bar up to your upper abs. Pause, then return the bar back to the starting position.

93 Back

Inverted Row

START

Grab a stationary bar with an overhand, shoulder-width grip. Your arms should be straight and your body should form a straight line from your shoulders to your ankles.

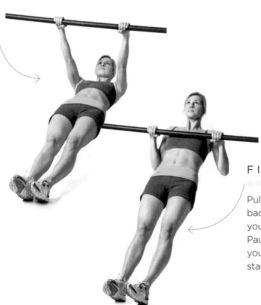

FINISH

Pull your shoulder blades back and lift your body until your chest touches the bar. Pause, then slowly lower your body back to the starting position.

45-Degree Cable Row

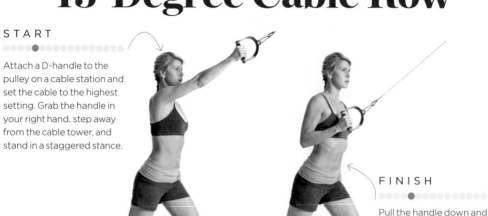

START

Attach a D-handle to the pulley on a cable station and set the cable to the highest setting. Grab the handle in your right hand, step away from the cable tower, and stand in a staggered stance.

FINISH

Pull the handle down and towards your right side by squeezing your shoulder blade back. Pause, then return to the starting position. Perform all reps, switch hands, and repeat.

Resistance Band Row

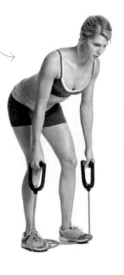
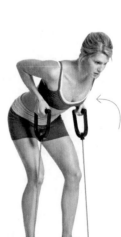

START

Grab a resistance band and step on it with one foot (use both feet for more resistance). Hold the band in each hand at arm's length, about shoulder-width apart, and then bend at your hips and lower your torso until it's almost parallel to the floor. Your knees should be slightly bent and your lower back naturally arched.

FINISH

Squeeze your shoulder blades together and pull the band up to your upper abs. Pause, then return the bar back to the starting position.

Row with Rotation

START

Grab a dumbbell with an overhand grip in your right hand. Hold the dumbbell at arm's length, then bend at your hips and lower your torso until it's almost parallel to the floor. Your knees should be slightly bent, your lower back naturally arched, and your other hand placed on your hip.

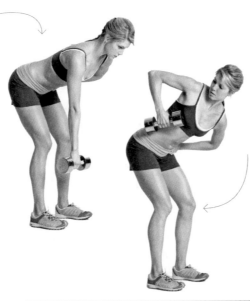

FINISH

Squeeze your shoulder blades back and then pull the dumbbell up to the sides of your torso and rotate your torso upwards. Pause, then return to the starting position. Complete all prescribed reps, switch arms, and repeat.

95 Back

Dumbbell Row

START

Grab a pair of dumbbells with an overhand grip with your hands about shoulder-width apart. Hold the dumbbells at arm's length, and then bend at your hips and lower your torso until it's almost parallel to the floor. Your knees should be slightly bent and your lower back naturally arched.

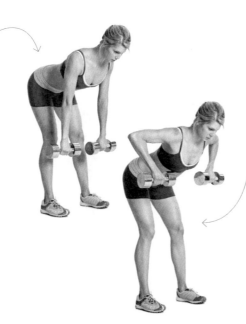

FINISH

Squeeze your shoulder blades together and pull the dumbbells up to the sides of your torso. Pause, then return to the starting position.

One-Arm Row

START

Grab a dumbbell in your right hand. Push your hips back and bend over until your torso is almost parallel to the floor. Place your left hand on a bench in front of your body. Your right arm should hang at arm's length with your palm facing your other arm.

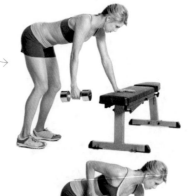

FINISH

Keeping your elbow close to your body, pull the dumbbell up to your chest by squeezing your shoulder blade back. Pause, then lower back to the starting position. Complete all prescribed reps, then switch arms and repeat.

Split-Stance Cable Row

START

Attach a D-handle to the pulley on a cable station and set the cable to about chest height. Grab the handle in your right hand, step away from the cable tower, and stand in a staggered stance.

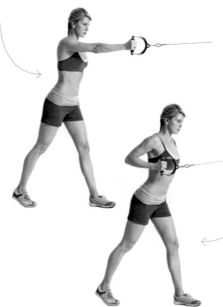

FINISH

Pull the handle towards your right side by squeezing your shoulder blade back. Pause, then return to the starting position. Perform all reps, switch hands, and repeat.

Band Pull-Apart

START

Grab a resistance band in both hands and hold the ends a little more than shoulder-width apart. Raise your arms so that the band is at arm's length in front of your chest.

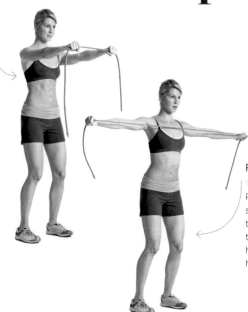

FINISH

Pull each end of the band and squeeze your shoulder blades together. Imagine you are trying to snap the band in half. Pause, then return your hands to the starting position.

97 Back

Resistance Band Pulldown

START

Loop one end of a large resistance band around a chin-up bar and then pull it through the other end of the band. Grab it with both hands about shoulder-width apart and your arms straight.

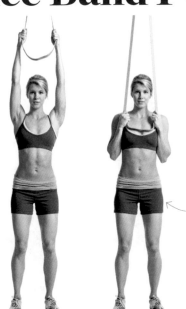

FINISH

Squeeze your shoulder blades down and back, and pull each hand to the side of your chest. Pause, then return to the starting position.

Lat Pulldown

START

Sit at a lat pulldown station and grab the bar with an overhand grip that's just beyond shoulder width. Your arms should be completely straight and your torso should be upright.

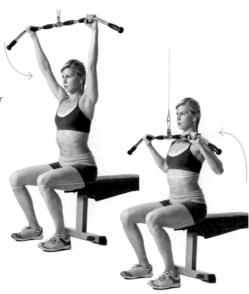

FINISH

Pull your shoulder blades down and back, and bring the bar to your chest. Pause, then return to the starting position.

Mixed-Grip Pulldown

START

Attach a bar to a lat pulldown station and grab the bar with a mixed grip – one hand over, the other under. Kneel on the floor so that your body forms a straight line from your shoulders to your knees.

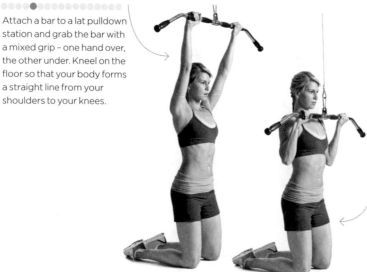

FINISH

Squeeze your shoulder blades down and back, then bring the bar to your chest.

Assisted Chin-Up

START

Loop one end of a large resistance band around a chin-up bar and then pull it through the other end of the band. Grab the bar with a shoulder-width, underhand grip. Place your knees in the loop of the band and hang at arm's length.

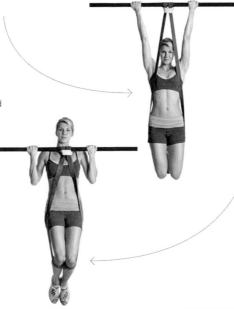

FINISH

Perform a chin-up by pulling your chest up to the bar. Once your chest touches the bar, pause, then lower your body back to the starting position.

99 Back

Negative Chin-up

START

Set a bench under a chin-up bar, step up on the bench, and grasp the bar using a shoulder-width grip. From the bench, jump up so that your chest is touching the bar.

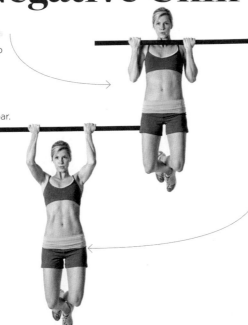

FINISH

Cross your ankles behind you, and try to take 5 seconds to lower your body until your arms are straight. If that's too hard, lower yourself as slowly as you can. Jump back up to the start and repeat.

Arm moves

FIGHT OFF ARM FLAB AND BUILD LEAN, SEXY BICEPS AND TRICEPS

Overhead Tricep Extension

START

Grab a dumbbell and stand tall with your feet shoulder-width apart. Hold the dumbbell at arm's length above your head, your palms facing each other.

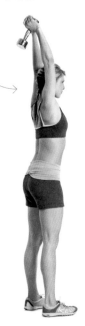
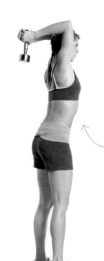

FINISH

Without moving your upper arms, lower the dumbbell behind your head. Pause, then straighten your arms to return the dumbbell to the starting position

101
Arms

Bicep Curl

START

Grab a pair of dumbbells and let them hang at arm's length next to your sides with your palms facing forwards.

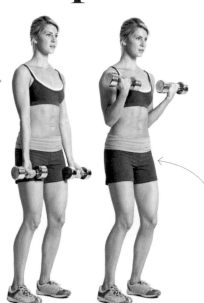

FINISH

Without moving your upper arms, bend your elbows and curl the dumbbells as close to your shoulders as you can. Pause, then lower the weights back to the starting position.

Dip

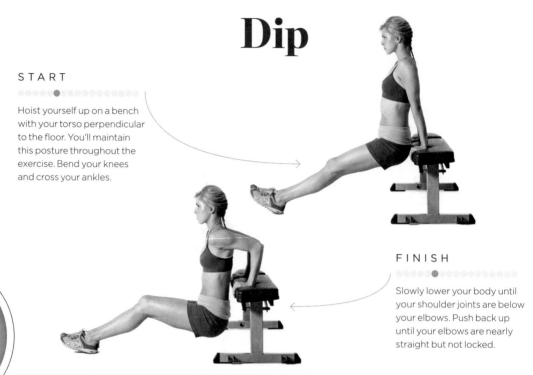

START

Hoist yourself up on a bench with your torso perpendicular to the floor. You'll maintain this posture throughout the exercise. Bend your knees and cross your ankles.

FINISH

Slowly lower your body until your shoulder joints are below your elbows. Push back up until your elbows are nearly straight but not locked.

Dumbbell Pullover

START

Grab a dumbbell and lie face up on a bench so only your head, neck, and upper back are supported by it. Your feet will be flat on the floor. (If this is too difficult, lie on top of the entire bench). Hold the dumbbell straight over your chin with your arms extended.

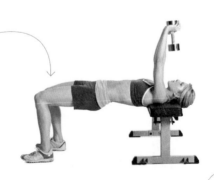

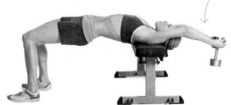

FINISH

Without changing the angle of your elbows, slowly lower the dumbbell back beyond your head until your upper arms are in line with your body or parallel to the floor. Pause, then slowly raise the dumbbells back to the starting position.

Resistance Band Curl

START

Stand on one end of a resistance band with both feet about shoulder-width apart. Grab the other end of the band with your hands about shoulder-width apart and your arms at your sides.

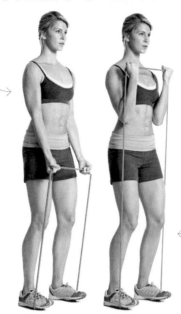

FINISH

Without moving your upper arms, bend your arms and pull the band as close to your shoulders as you can. Pause, then lower the band to the starting position.

103
Arms

Band Overhead Press

START

Loop one end of a large resistance band around a chin-up bar (or a secure object) and then pull it through the other end of the band. Grab the band with each hand and your back to the anchor point. Stand in a staggered stance, one foot in front of the other. Hold the band behind your head, your elbows pointing forward and bent 90 degrees.

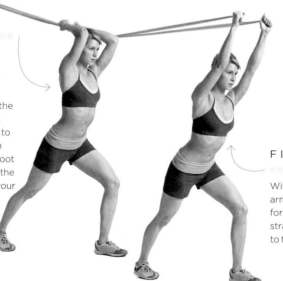

FINISH

Without moving your upper arms, push your forearms forwards until your arms are straight. Pause, then return to the starting position.

Chapter Seven

Shoulder moves

LOOK GREAT IN ANY VEST TOP
OR T-SHIRT BY TARGETING
THESE MUSCLES

Wall Slide

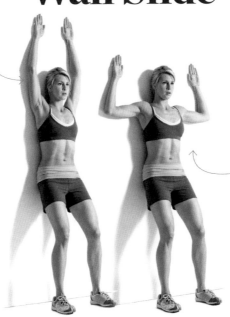

START

Lean your head, upper back, and bum against the wall. Place your hands and arms against the wall in the "high-five" position, your elbows bent 90 degrees and your upper arms at shoulder height. Hold for 1 second. Don't allow your head, upper back, or bum to lose contact with the wall.

FINISH

Keeping your elbows, wrists, and hands pressed into the wall, slide your elbows down toward your sides as far as you can. Squeeze your shoulder blades together. Slide your arms back up the wall as high as you can while keeping your hands against it. Lower and repeat.

105 Shoulders

Lateral Shoulder Raise

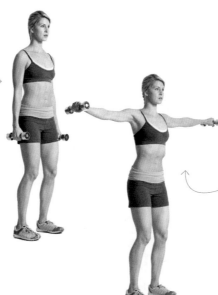

START

Grab a pair of dumbbells and let them hang at arm's length next to your sides. Stand tall and make sure your palms are facing your body.

FINISH

Keeping your elbows slightly bent, raise your arms straight out to the sides until they're at shoulder level. Pause, then lower the weights back to the starting position.

Lateral Raise

START

Grab a pair of dumbbells
and bend forward at your
hips until your back is nearly
parallel to the floor. Your arms
should hang straight down
from your shoulders with your
elbows slightly bent.

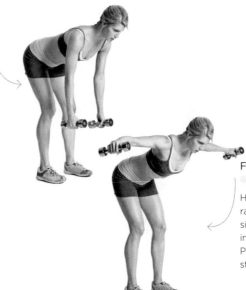

FINISH

Hold your body still and
raise your arms out to the
sides until your hands are
in line with your shoulders.
Pause, then return to the
starting position.

T Raise

START

Lie chest down on an
adjustable bench set to a
low incline. Your arms should
hang straight down from your
shoulders, and your palms
should be facing each other.

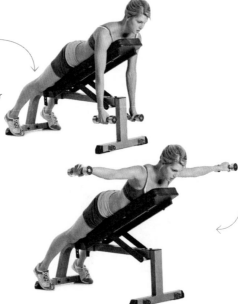

FINISH

Raise your arms straight out
to your sides until they're in
line with your body. At the top
of the movement, your arms
and torso should form a T.
Pause, then lower your arms
back to the starting position.

Y Raise

START

Lie chest down on an adjustable bench set to a low incline. Your arms should hang straight down from your shoulders, and your palms should be facing each other.

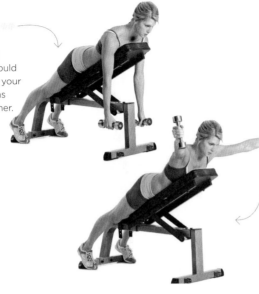

FINISH

Raise your arms at a 30-degree angle to your body until they are in line with your body. At the top of the movement, your arms and torso should form a Y. Pause, then lower back to the starting position.

I Raise

START

Lie chest down on an adjustable bench set to a low incline. Your arms should hang straight down from your shoulders, and your palms should be facing each other.

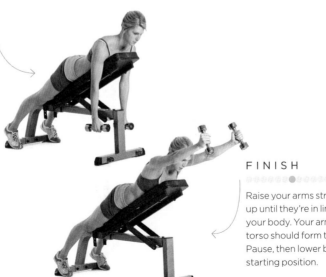

FINISH

Raise your arms straight up until they're in line with your body. Your arms and torso should form the letter I. Pause, then lower back to the starting position.

Overhead Press

START

Grab a pair of dumbbells and hold them just in front of your shoulders with your palms facing each other.

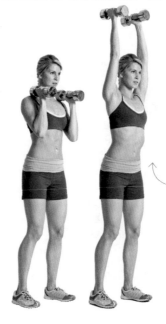

FINISH

Press the weight over-head until your arms are completely straight. Pause, then slowly lower the dumbbells back to the starting position.

One-Arm Overhead Press

START

Grab one dumbbell with one hand and hold it just outside your shoulder with your palm facing your head.

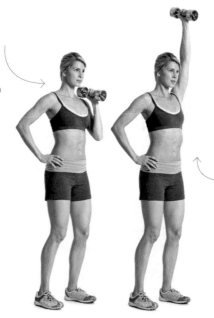

FINISH

Press the weight overhead until your arm is completely straight. Pause, then slowly lower the dumbbell back to the starting position. Complete all reps, then swap the dumbbell to your other hand and repeat.

Shoulder Press With Twist

START

Grab a pair of dumbbells and hold them just in front of your shoulders with your palms facing each other.

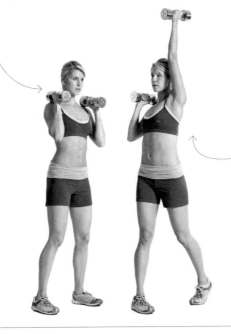

FINISH

Rotate your torso to the right, pivot your left foot, and press the dumbbell in your left hand overhead. Reverse the movement and return to the starting position. Rotate to the left and press the dumbbell in your right hand overhead. Continue alternating back and forth.

109
Shoulders

Barbell Shoulder Press

START

Grab a barbell with an overhand grip that's just beyond shoulder width and hold it at shoulder level in front of your body. Stand with your feet shoulder-width apart and your knees slightly bent.

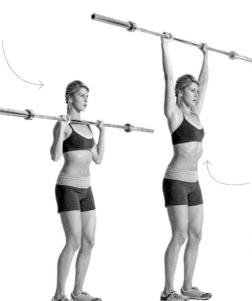

FINISH

Push the barbell straight overhead, while keeping your torso upright. Pause, then lower the bar back to the starting position.

Chapter Eight

Total-body moves

THE BEST WAY TO BLAST FAT IS WITH MOVES THAT WORK ALL OF YOUR MUSCLES

Jumping Jack

START

Stand with your feet together and your hands at your sides.

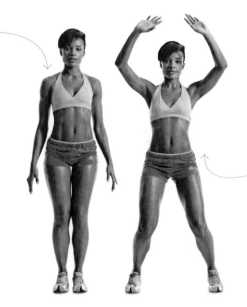

FINISH

Simultaneously raise your arms above your head and jump your feet out to the sides. Immediately, reverse the movement and jump back to the starting position. Repeat for all reps.

Band Curl to Squat to Press

**111
Total body**

START

Stand on a resistance band with your feet shoulder-width apart. Grab the ends of the band with your hands about shoulder-width apart and your arms at your sides. Without moving your upper arms, bend your arms and pull the band as close to your shoulders as you can. Pause, then lower the band to the starting position.

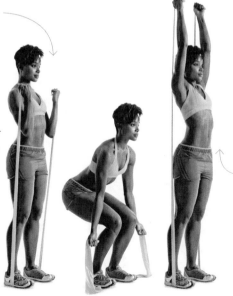

FINISH

Push your hips back and squat down until your upper thighs are at least parallel to the floor. Immediately, explode upwards, stand up, and press the band overhead. That's 1 rep.

Squat Thrust

START

Stand with your feet shoulder-width apart and your arms at your sides. Push your hips back, bend your knees, and lower your body as deep as you can into a squat.

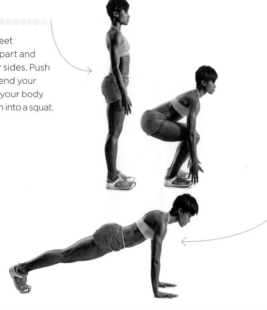

FINISH

Place your hands on the floor, and kick your legs backwards into a press-up position. Kick your legs back to the squat position. Stand up and jump. That's 1 rep.

Squat to Stand

START

Stand tall with your legs straight, feet shoulder-width apart. Bend over and grab your toes (if you need to bend your knees, you can.) Without letting go of your toes, lower your body into a squat as you raise your chest and shoulders up.

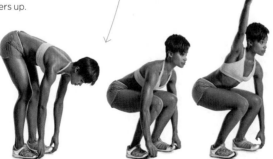

FINISH

Staying in the squat position, raise your right arm up high and wide. Then raise your left arm. Now stand up.

Goblet Squat to Press

START

Hold a dumbbell vertically next to your chest, with both hands cupping the dumbbell head. Push your hips back and lower your body into a squat until your upper thighs are at least parallel to the floor. Your elbows should brush the insides of your knees in the bottom position.

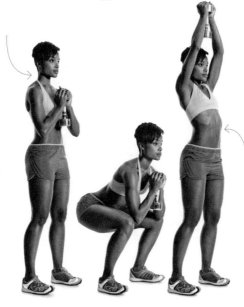

FINISH

Pause, then press your body back up and press the dumbbell overhead. Lower the dumbbell back to the starting position.

Dumbbell Squat Thrust

START

Stand with your feet shoulder-width apart and your arms at your sides holding a pair of dumbbells. Push your hips back, bend your knees, and lower your body as deep as you can into a squat

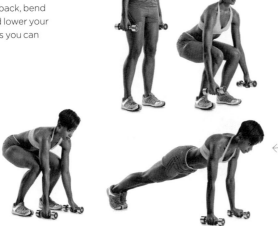

FINISH

Place the dumbbells on the floor, then kick your legs backward into a press-up position. Kick your legs back to the squat position. Stand up and jump. That's 1 rep.

113 Total body

Dumbbell Push Press

114
Total body

START

Grab a pair of dumbbells and hold them just outside your shoulders with your palms facing each other. Bend your knees and lower your body into a half squat

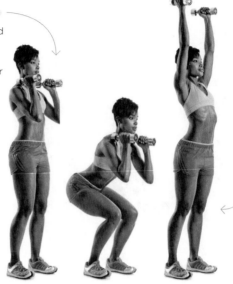

FINISH

Press the weight overhead as you stand up tall and explode upwards, pressing through your heels. Pause, then slowly lower the dumbbells back to the starting position.

Dumbbell Snatch

START

Place a dumbbell on the floor and stand over it with your feet wider than shoulder-width apart. Bend at your hips and knees, and squat down until you can grab the dumbbell with one hand, without rounding your upper back

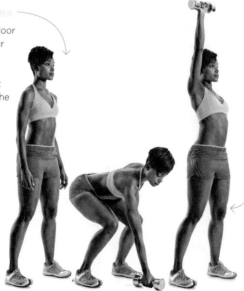

FINISH

Keeping the dumbbell close to your body, pull the dumbbell upward and try to throw it at the ceiling without letting go. As you raise the dumbbell, your forearm should rotate up and back, until your arm is straight and your palm is facing forward. Pause and then lower the weight back down to the starting position.

Dumbbell Swing

START

Grab a dumbbell (or kettlebell) with an overhand grip and hold it with one hand in front of your waist at arm's length. Set your feet slightly wider than shoulder-width apart. Keeping your lower back slightly arched, bend at your hips and knees, and lower your torso until it forms a 45-degree angle to the floor. Now swing the dumbbell backwards between your legs.

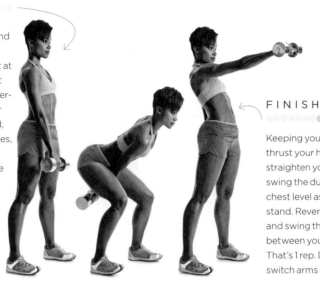

FINISH

Keeping your arm straight, thrust your hips forward, straighten your knees, and swing the dumbbell up to chest level as you rise to stand. Reverse the movement and swing the dumbbell back between your legs again. That's 1 rep. Do all reps, then switch arms and repeat.

Band Squat and Press

START

Loop one end of a large resistance band around a secure object and then pull it through the other end of the band. Grab the band with each hand and your back to the anchor point. Stand with your feet shoulder-width apart. Squat down holding the band behind your head, your elbows pointing forward and bent 90 degrees.

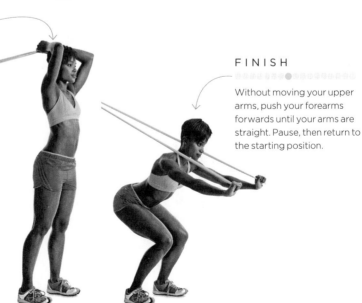

FINISH

Without moving your upper arms, push your forearms forwards until your arms are straight. Pause, then return to the starting position.

115
Total body

Dumbbell Clean

START

Squat over a pair of
dumbbells and grab them
with an overhand grip. Stand
and lift both weights up to
chest height.

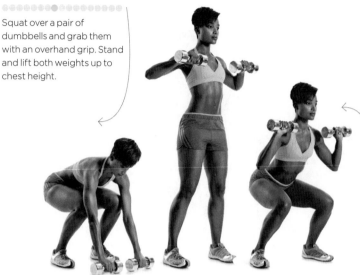

FINISH

Quickly drop underneath
the weights and "catch"
them on your shoulders,
with your elbows high. Drop
your elbows, keeping the
dumbbells at shoulder level.

Dumbbell High Pull

START

Grab a pair of dumbbells with
an overhand grip and hold
them just below knee height.

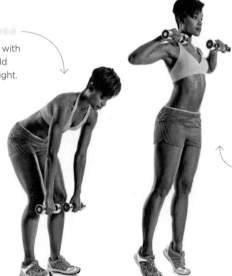

FINISH

Explosively pull the
dumbbells upwards, rise
onto your toes, and bend
your elbows as you bring
the weights up to shoulder
height. Return to the
starting position.

Lunge and Cable Row

START

Attach a D-handle at hip height to a cable station. Grab the handle and step away from the tower until your arm is extended in front of your body. Step backward into a lunge and lower your body until your front knee is bent 90 degrees.

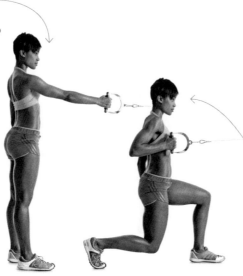

FINISH

Pause, row the cable to the side of your chest, and then return to the starting position. Perform all reps, and then switch arms and repeat the process, stepping back with your other leg.

117
Total body

Dumbbell Jump Shrug

START

Grab a pair of dumbbells and let them hang at arm's length with your palms facing each other. Push your hips back, slightly bend your knees, and lower the dumbbells until they are just below your knees

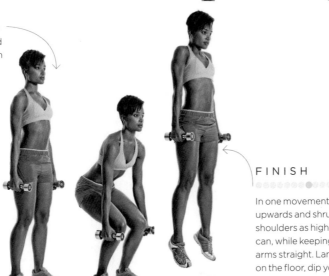

FINISH

In one movement, explode upwards and shrug your shoulders as high as you can, while keeping your arms straight. Land softly on the floor, dip your knees, and repeat

Lunge with Bicep Curl

118
Total body

START

Grab a pair of dumbbells and hold them at arm's length next to your sides, your palms facing each other. Stand tall with your feet hip-width apart. Step forward with your right leg and lower your body until your front knee is bent 90 degrees. At the same time as you lunge, curl both dumbbells up to your shoulders

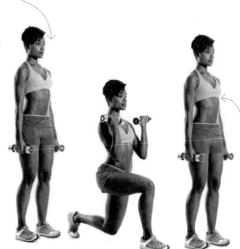

FINISH

Lower the dumbbells, and then return to the starting position. Step forward with the other leg and repeat. Continue alternating legs.

Lunge and Reach

START

Stand tall with your arms hanging at your sides. Brace your core and hold it that way. Lunge back with your right leg, lowering your body until your left knee is bent at least 90 degrees.

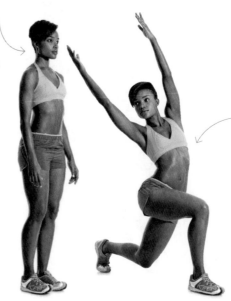

FINISH

As you lunge, reach back with both hands over your shoulders and to the left. Reverse the movement back to the starting position. Complete the prescribed number of repetitions with your left leg, then step back with your left leg and reach over your right shoulder for the same number of reps. Keep your torso upright for the entire movement.

Side Lunge with Bicep Curl

START

Hold a pair of dumbbells at arm's length with your palms facing forwards and your feet shoulder-width apart. Lift your left foot and take a step to the left as you push your hips backward and lower your body by dropping your hips and bending your left knee. Your right leg should remain straight in the "bottom" position of the lunge.

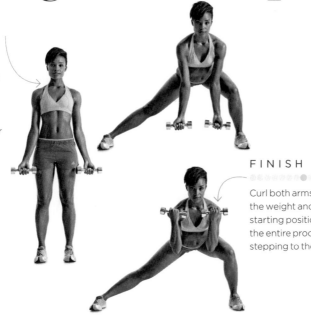

FINISH

Curl both arms up. Lower the weight and return to the starting position. Repeat the entire process, this time stepping to the right.

Dumbbell Renegade Crawl

START

Grab a dumbbell with each hand and get into the standard press-up position. Lower your body to the floor, pause, then push yourself back up. Once you're back in the starting position, lift the dumbbell in your right hand to the right side of your chest.

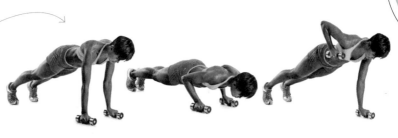

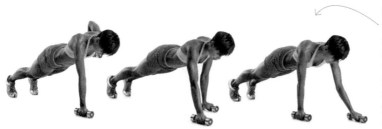

FINISH

Lower the dumbbell and repeat with your left hand. "Walk" each hand one step forward, still holding the dumbbells, and follow with your feet so you're back in the starting position. That's 1 rep.

119
Total body

Squat and Cable Row

START

Attach a D-handle at hip height to a cable station. Grab the handle with one hand and step away from the tower until your arm is extended in front of your body.

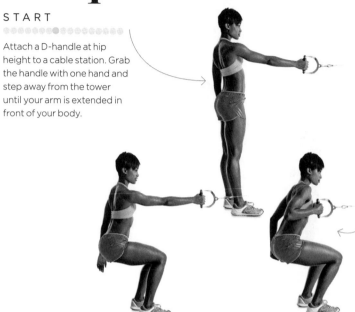

FINISH

Push your hips back and lower your body into a squat until your thighs are at least parallel to the floor. Pause, row the cable to the side of your chest, and then return to the starting position. Perform all reps, then switch arms and repeat the process.

Split Squat and Press

START

Grab a bar with an overhand grip around shoulder-width apart and hold it at shoulder height. Stand in a staggered stance with your right foot in front of your left and your front knee slightly bent.

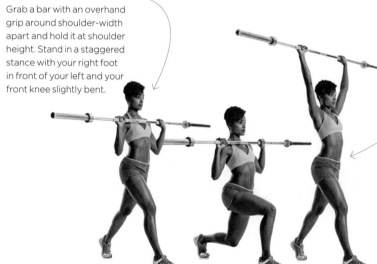

FINISH

Lower your body as far as you can, or until your back knee nearly touches the floor. Push yourself back up to the starting position. As you stand up, press the bar overhead. Return to the starting position and repeat.

Squat to Overhead Press

START

Grab a pair of dumbbells and hold them next to your shoulders, your palms facing each other. Stand tall with your feet shoulder-width apart. Lower your body until the tops of your thighs are at least parallel to the floor.

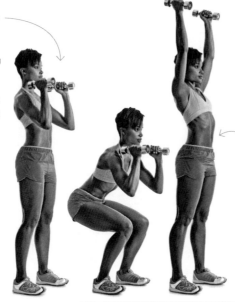

FINISH

Push your body back to standing position as you press the dumbbell directly over your shoulders. Lower the dumbbells back to the starting position.

Band Squat and Stand

START

Grab the ends of a resistance band in each hand and stand on the middle with your feet shoulder-width apart. Hold the ends at shoulder height with your palms facing away from your body.

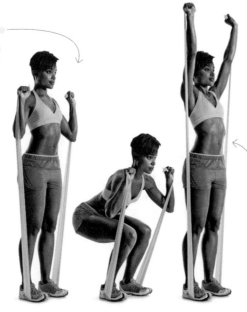

FINISH

Push your hips back, bend your knees, and lower your body into a squat until your upper thighs are at least parallel to the floor. Press back up to the starting position, pressing your arms overhead until your arms are straight. Lower your arms. That's 1 rep.

121
Total body

Inchworm

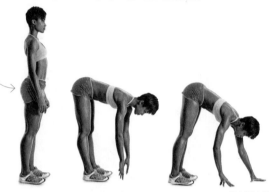

START

Stand tall with your legs straight. Bend at your hips. Begin "walking" forwards with your hands.

FINISH

Keeping your legs straight, walk your hands forwards as far as you can without allowing your hips to sag. Now walk your feet towards your hands. That's 1 rep

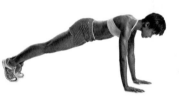

Kettlebell Windmill

START

Stand with your feet wider than hip-width apart, and hold the kettlebell in your left hand. Raise it next to your left shoulder then press it overhead.

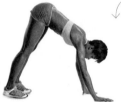

FINISH

Rotate your chest to the left and look up at the kettlebell as you try to touch your right hand to your right foot. Pause, then return to the starting position, keeping your left arm extended. Do the prescribed number of reps before lowering the weight, then repeat on the other side.

Band Squat and Row

START

Loop one end of a large resistance band around a secure object and pull it through the other end of the band. Grab the handle and step away from the anchor point until your arm is extended in front of your body.

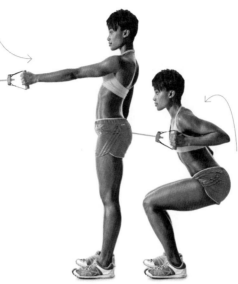

FINISH

Push your hips back and lower your body into a squat until your thighs are at least parallel to the floor. Pause, then row the band to the side of your chest and return to the starting position. Perform all reps, then switch arms and repeat the process.

One-Arm Farmer's Carry

START

Hold a dumbbell in your right hand straight above your shoulder with your arm completely straight and your palm facing out

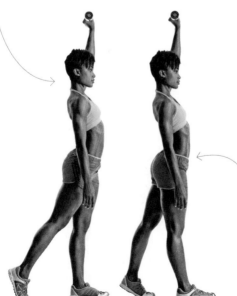

FINISH

Keeping your arm locked in this position, walk forward the prescribed number of steps while maintaining your upright posture. Complete all reps, switch arms, and repeat.

123
Total body

Lunge to Curl to Press

START

Hold a pair of dumbbells at arm's length at your sides. Step forward with your right leg and lower your body until your front knee is bent at least 90 degrees. Curl the dumbbells to your chest as you sink down, and as you rise, rotate your wrists so that your palms face forward.

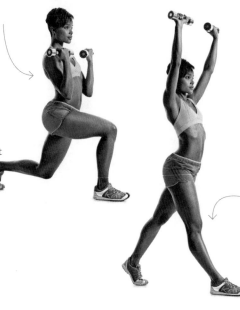

FINISH

Press the dumbbells overhead when you are in the standing position. Return your arms to the starting position. Repeat, this time stepping forward with your left leg.

124
Total body

Step-up and Press

START

Grab a dumbbell and hold it in your right hand, with your arm bent 90 degrees, so that the dumbbell is just above your shoulder. Your palm should be in line with your shoulder. Place your left foot on a box or step that's about knee height

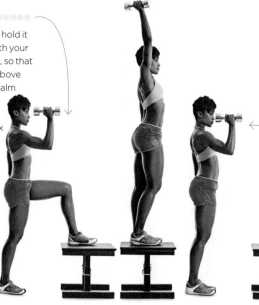

FINISH

Push down with your left heel, and step up onto the box as you push the dumbbell straight above your right shoulder. Lower your arm and step back down. Do all of the prescribed repetitions with your left foot lifting you onto the box and the weight in your right hand. Switch arms and legs, and repeat.

Lunge and One-Arm Press

START

Stand with your feet slightly closer than shoulder-width apart. Grab a dumbbell with your right hand and hold it next to your right shoulder, your palm facing in.

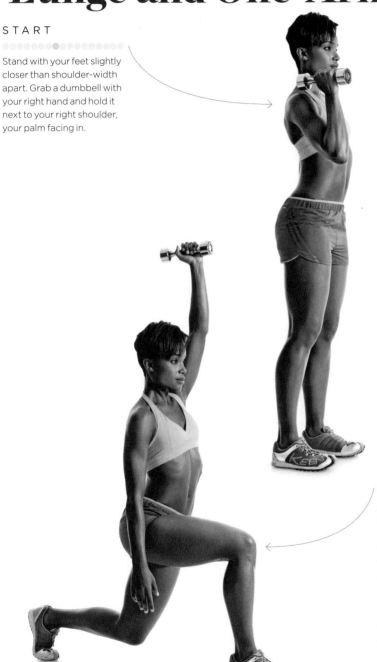

125
Total body

FINISH

Step backwards with your right leg and lower your body into a reverse lunge as you simultaneously press the dumbbell straight above your shoulder. Rise back up to return to the starting position, lower the dumbbell as you do so. That's 1 rep. Complete all your reps, then switch arms and legs and repeat.

Chapter Nine

Lower-body moves

BLAST AWAY CELLULITE,
TIGHTEN YOUR BUM AND FIT
INTO YOUR SKINNY JEANS

Barbell Squat

START

Hold a barbell across your upper back with an overhand grip and your feet shoulder-width apart.

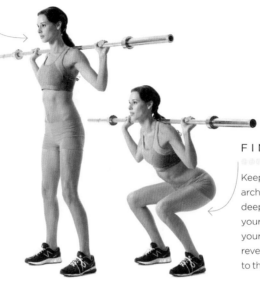

FINISH

Keeping your lower back arched, lower your body as deep as you can by pushing your hips back and bending your knees. Pause, then reverse the movement back to the starting position.

Bodyweight Squat

START

Stand tall with your feet shoulder-width apart and place your fingers on the back of your head.

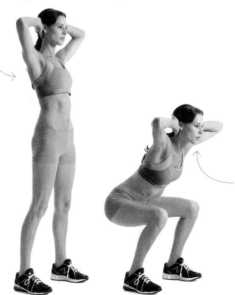

FINISH

Pull your shoulders and elbows back, and lower your body as far as you can by pushing your hips back and bending your knees. Pause, then push yourself back to the starting position.

127
Lower body

Dumbbell Front Squat

START

Stand with your feet shoulder-width apart. Hold a pair of dumbbells so that your palms are facing each other, and rest one of the dumbbell heads on the meatiest part of each shoulder. Keep your body as upright as you can at all times, as your upper arms remain parallel to the floor.

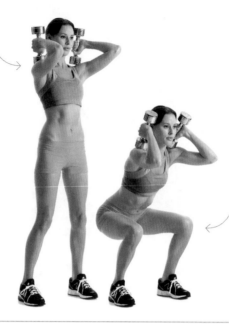

FINISH

Brace your abs and lower your body as far as you can by pushing your hips back and bending your knees. Pause, then push yourself back to the starting position.

Sumo Front Squat

START

Grab a dumbbell in one hand and hold it at arm's length in front of your waist. Set your feet about twice shoulder-width with your toes turned slightly outward.

FINISH

Push your hips back and lower your body into a squat until your upper thighs are at least parallel to the floor. Pause, then press your body back up to the starting position, keeping your back upright and straight at all times.

Squat Jump

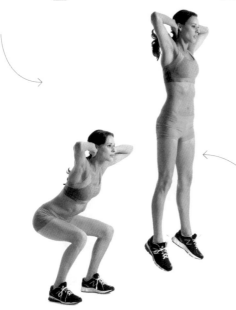

START

Place your fingers on the back of your head and pull your elbows back so that they're in line with your body. Dip your knees in preparation to leap.

FINISH

Explosively jump as high as you can, raising your arms up in the air as you jump. When you land, immediately squat down and jump again.

Dumbbell Split Squat

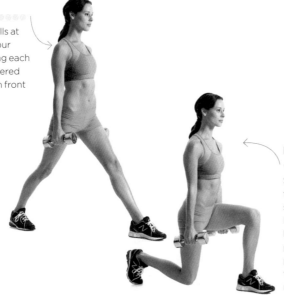

START

Hold a pair of dumbbells at arm's length next to your sides, your palms facing each other. Stand in a staggered stance, your left foot in front of your right.

FINISH

Slowly lower your body as far as you can. Your rear knee should nearly touch the floor. Pause, then push yourself back up to the starting position. Complete the prescribed number of reps, then do the same number of reps with your right foot in front of your left.

129
Lower body

FLAT BELLY WORKOUTS

Dumbbell Squat

START

Hold a pair of dumbbells at arm's length next to your sides, your palms facing each other.

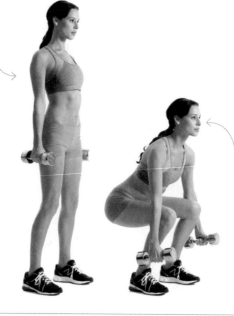

FINISH

Brace your abs, and lower your body as far as you can by pushing your hips back and bending your knees. Pause, then push back up to the starting position.

Band Lateral Squat

START

Place both legs between a mini resistance band and position the band just below your knees.

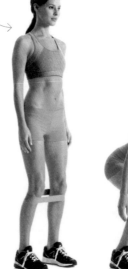

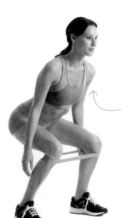

FINISH

Take a side step to the right and push your hips back and bend your knees so you lower your body into a squat. Stand back up. That's 1 rep. Complete the prescribed number of reps, then sidestep to your left for the same number of reps. That's 1 set.

Goblet Squat

131
Lower body

START

Hold a dumbbell vertically next to your chest, with both hands cupping the dumbbell head.

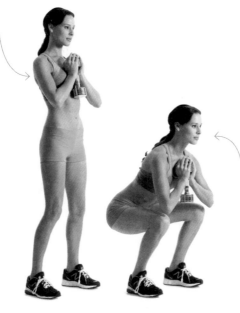

FINISH

Push your hips back and lower your body into a squat until your upper thighs are at least parallel to the floor. Your elbows should brush the insides of your knees in the bottom position. Pause, then press your body back up to the starting position.

Overhead Split Squat

START

Hold a pair of dumbbells directly over your shoulders, with your arms completely straight. Squeeze your abs tight for the entire exercise. Stand in a staggered stance, your left foot in front of your right foot.

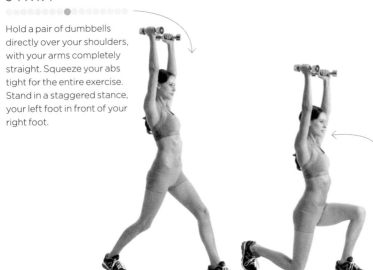

FINISH

Push your hips back and bend your knees so you lower your body into a squat. Pause, then push yourself back up to the starting position. Perform the prescribed number of reps, and then do the same number of reps with your right foot in front of your left.

Single-Leg Squat

START

Stand on your left leg in front of a bench or box that's about knee height. Hold your arms straight out in front of you.

FINISH

Balancing on your left foot, bend your left knee and slowly lower your body until your right heel lightly touches the floor. Pause, then push yourself up. Complete the prescribed number of reps with your left leg, then immediately do the same number with your right. If this is too hard, lower your body as far as you can, pause, then press back up.

Elevated Rear Split Squat

START

Hold a pair of dumbbells at arm's length next to your sides, your palms facing each other. Stand in a staggered stance with your left foot in front of your right, and place the instep of your back foot on a bench

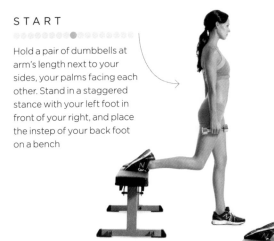

FINISH

Lower your body as far as you can, pause, then push your body back up to the starting position. Do all reps with your left foot forward, then do the same number with your right foot in front of your left.

Calf Raise

START

Grab a dumbbell in your right hand and stand on a step or weight plate. Cross your left foot behind your right ankle, and balance your body on the ball of your right foot, with your right heel on the floor or hanging off the step.

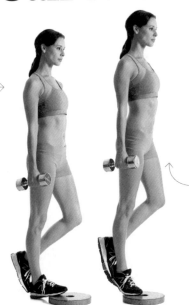

FINISH

Lift your right heel as high as you can. Pause, then lower and repeat. Complete the prescribed number of reps with your right leg, then do the same number with your left leg while holding the dumbbell in your left hand.

133
Lower body

Skater Jump

START

Stand on your right foot your knee slightly bent, and place your left foot just behind your right ankle. Lower your body into a squat. Bound to the left foot by jumping off your right foot.

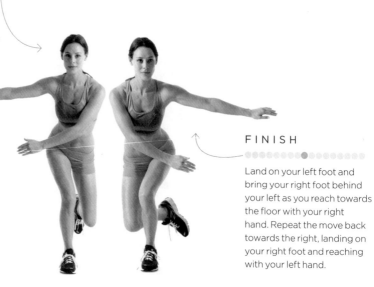

FINISH

Land on your left foot and bring your right foot behind your left as you reach towards the floor with your right hand. Repeat the move back towards the right, landing on your right foot and reaching with your left hand.

Box Jump

START

Stand in front of a sturdy, secure box that's high enough so that you have to jump with great effort in order to land on top of it. Dip your knees, and then explosively jump into the air

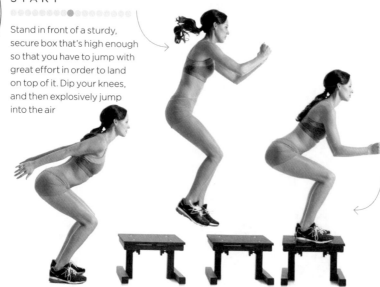

FINISH

Land on the top of the box with a "soft" landing by ensuring you bend your knees to absorb the impact. Step down and return to the starting position. Once you've mastered this you can make it more challenging by holding a dumbbell in each hand

Split Jump

START

Stand in a staggered stance, your left foot in front of your right foot. Lower your body as far as you can. Quickly jump into the air with enough force that you can switch the direction of your feet in the air

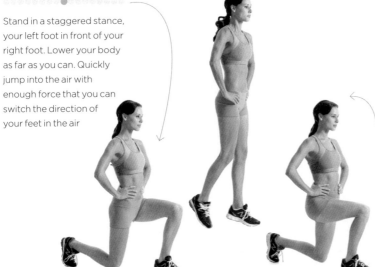

FINISH

Land with your right foot in front of your left. Continue alternating back and forth with each repetition. Once you've mastered this you can make it more challenging by holding a dumbbell in each hand

Jump Lunges

START

Hold a pair of dumbbells at arm's length next to your sides, your palms facing each other. Stand in a staggered stance, your left foot in front of your right. Lower your body as far as you can, or until your rear knee nearly touches the floor.

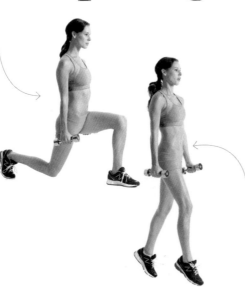

FINISH

Quickly jump into the air with enough force that you can scissor-kick your legs so you land with the opposite leg forward. Repeat, alternating back and forth with each repetition.

135
Lower body

Bodyweight Lunge

START

Place your hands on your hips, pull your shoulders back, and stand as tall as you can.

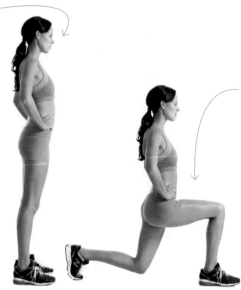

FINISH

Step forwards with your right leg and slowly lower your body until your front knee is bent at least 90 degrees. Pause, then push yourself to the starting position as quickly as you can. Complete the prescribed number of reps with your right leg, then do the same number with your left leg. For a greater challenge hold a dumbbell in each hand, arms hanging at your sides, while you do this.

Cross-Behind Lunge

START

Grab a pair of dumbbells and hold them at arm's length at your sides, your palms facing each other.

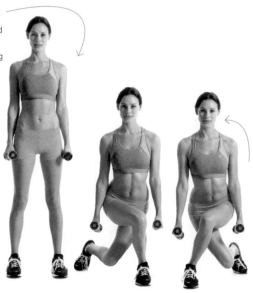

FINISH

Step forwards and to the side so that your lead foot ends up in front of your back foot (like a curtsy).Lower your body until your front knee is bent 90 degrees. Pause, then return to the starting position and repeat with your other leg.

Goblet Lunge

START

Hold a dumbbell vertically next to your chest, with both hands cupping the dumbbell head.

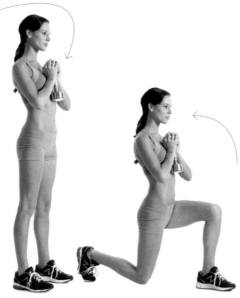

FINISH

Step backwards with your left leg. Lower your body into a lunge until your front leg is bent 90 degrees. Pause, then return to the starting position. Do all your reps and then repeat with your other leg.

Dumbbell Reverse Lunge

START

Grab a pair of dumbbells and hold them at arm's length next to your sides, your palms facing each other.

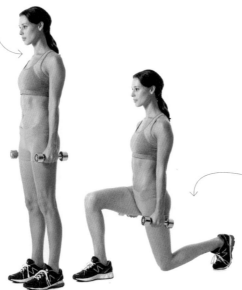

FINISH

Step backwards with your left leg. Lower your body into a lunge until your front leg is bent 90 degrees. Pause, then return to the starting position. Do all your reps and then repeat with your other leg

137
Lower body

Reverse Lunge and Rotate

START

Grab a dumbbell and hold it by the ends, just below your chin. Stand tall with your feet slightly less than shoulder-width apart.

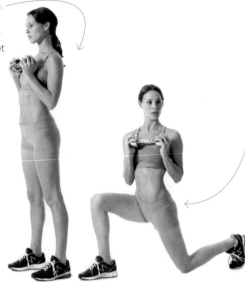

FINISH

Step backwards with your left leg and lower your body into a lunge until your front leg is bent 90 degrees. As you lunge, rotate your upper body towards the same side as the leg you're using to step backwards. Pause, then return to the starting position. Repeat on your other leg and continue alternating.

Lateral Bound with Pause

START

Stand with your hips pushed back and knees slightly bent. Dip your knees slightly, and then explosively hop off your right leg, swinging your arms and moving to your left.

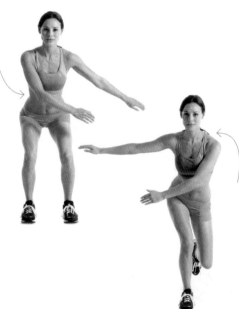

FINISH

Land on your left foot and pause until you remove all momentum. Then reverse the movement to the right. Back and forth once counts as 1 rep.

Step-ups

START

Grab a pair of dumbbells and hold them at arm's length at your sides. Stand in front of a step or bench and place your left foot firmly on the step. The step should be high enough that your knee is bent 90 degrees

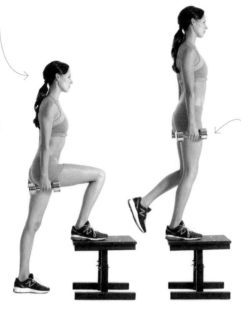

FINISH

Press your left heel into the step, and push your body up until your left leg is straight and you're standing on one leg on the step, keeping your right foot elevated. Lower your body down until your right foot touches the floor. That's 1 rep. Complete the prescribed number of reps with your left leg, then do the same number with your right.

Crossover Step-up

START

Grab a pair of dumbbells and stand with your left side next to a step at knee height. Place your right foot on the step.

FINISH

Press through your right heel and push your body up onto the step until both legs are straight. Lower your body back to the starting position. Perform the prescribed number of reps with your right leg, then switch to your left leg and repeat

139
Lower body

Romanian Deadlift

START

Grab a barbell with an overhand grip that's just beyond shoulder-width and hold it at arm's length in front of your hips. Your knees should be slightly bent and chest pushed out. This is the starting position.

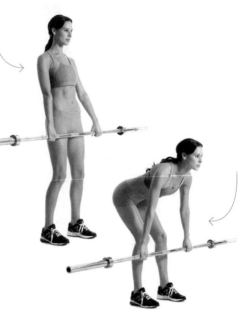

FINISH

Without changing the bend in your knees, bend at your hips and lower your torso until it's almost parallel to the floor. Pause, then raise your torso back to the starting position. If you don't have a barbell you can do the same move with a dumbbell in each hand.

Sumo Deadlift

START

Load a barbell and roll it up against your shins. Set your feet about twice shoulder-width apart with your toes pointed out an angle. Bend at your hips and knees, and grab the centre of the bar with an overhand grip and your hands about 12 inches apart.

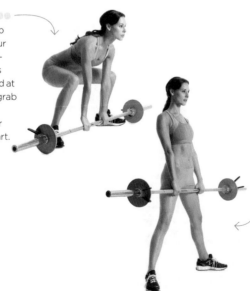

FINISH

Without allowing your lower back to round, stand up, thrust your hips forwards, squeezing your glutes. Pause, then lower the bar back to the floor while keeping it as close to your body as possible.

Snatch Grip Deadlift

START

Load a barbell and roll it up against your shins. Bend at your hips and knees, and grab the bar with an overhand grip that's about twice shoulder-width

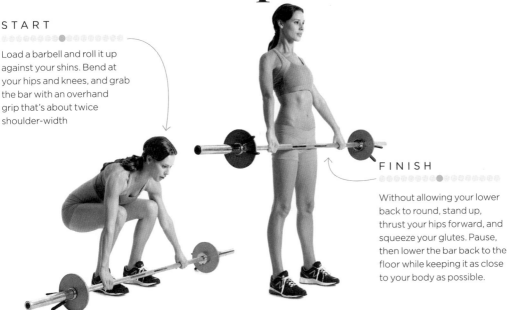

FINISH

Without allowing your lower back to round, stand up, thrust your hips forward, and squeeze your glutes. Pause, then lower the bar back to the floor while keeping it as close to your body as possible.

Dumbbell Deadlift

START

Set a pair of dumbbells on the floor in front of you. Bend at your hips and knees, and grab the dumbbells with an overhand grip.

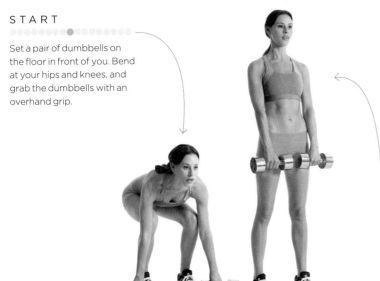

FINISH

Without allowing your lower back to round, stand up with the dumbbells and thrust your hips forward. Lower your body back down to the starting position.

141
Lower body

Hip Raise

START

Lie face up on the floor with your knees bent and your feet flat on the floor.

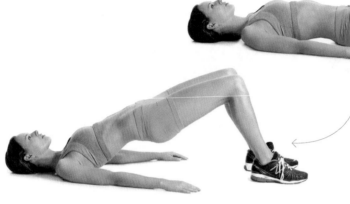

FINISH

Raise your hips so your body forms a straight line from your shoulders to your knees. Pause in the up position, then lower your body back to the starting position.

Barbell Hip Raise

START

Sit on the floor with your upper back against a stable bench, your knees bent and feet flat on the floor. Put a padded barbell across your hips and grab the barbell with an overhand grip, about shoulder-width apart.

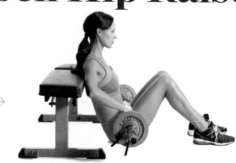

FINISH

Keeping your back against the bench and the barbell just below your pelvis, raise your hips – while squeezing your glutes – until your hips are in line with your body. Return to the starting position. Repeat.

Single-Leg Hip Raise

START

Lie face up on the floor with your right knee bent and your left leg straight. Raise your left leg until it's in line with your right thigh. Place your arms out to the side.

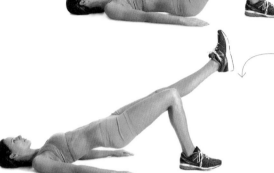

FINISH

Push your hips upwards, keeping your left leg elevated. Pause, then slowly lower your body and legs back to the starting position. Complete the prescribed number of reps with your left leg, then switch legs and do the same number with your right leg.

Side Lying Hip Abduction

START

Lie on the floor on your left side and loop a mini resistance band around your ankles. Put your right arm on your hip and prop your head up with your left arm.

143
Lower body

FINISH

Without moving any other part of your body, raise your right leg as high as you can. Your legs should remain straight. Pause, then return to the starting position. Do all reps, roll to your other side, and repeat.

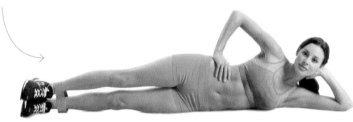

Lateral Lunge

START

Place your hands on your hips, pull your shoulders back, and stand as tall as you can.

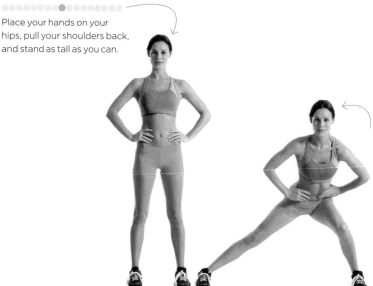

FINISH

Lift your left foot and take a big step to your left as you push your hips backward and lower your body by dropping your hips and bending your left knee. Pause, then quickly push yourself back to the starting position. For a greater challenge hold a dumbbell in each hand, arms hanging at your sides, while you do this.

Lateral Band Walk

START

Place both legs between a mini resistance band, and position the band just below your knees.

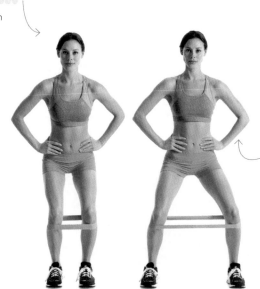

FINISH

Take small steps to your right for the prescribed number of reps. Sidestep back to your left for the same number of reps. That's 1 set.

Swiss Ball Leg Curl

START

Lie face up on the floor, and place your lower legs and heels on a Swiss ball. Push your hips up so that your body forms a straight line from shoulders to knees.

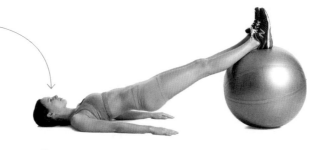

FINISH

Pull your heels toward your body and roll the ball as close as possible to your butt. Pause, then reverse the motion and roll the ball back until your body is in a straight line. Lower your hips to the floor and repeat.

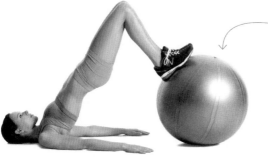

TRX Leg Curl

START

Lie face up on the floor and place both of your feet in the foot cradles of the TRX. Push your hips up so that your body forms a straight line from your shoulders to your knees.

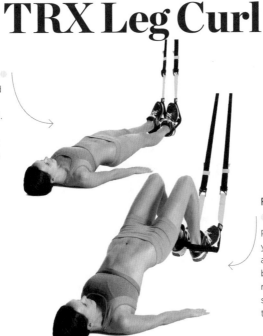

FINISH

Pull your heels towards your body so your feet are as close as possible to your bum. Pause, then reverse the motion until your body is in a straight line. Lower your hips to the floor and then repeat.

145
Lower body

Chapter Ten

Ab moves

UNLOCK THE POTENTIAL
OF YOUR BODY AND GET
A TIGHT, FLAT BELLY

Sit-up

START

Lie on your back with your knees bent and your feet flat on the floor. Place your fingertips behind your ears and pull your shoulder blades back so your elbows are out to the sides.

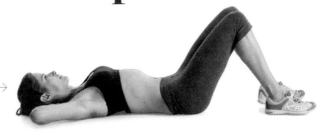

FINISH

Contract your abs and then raise your body up towards your knees. Pause, then slowly roll back down to the starting position.

Reverse Crunch

START

Lie face up on the floor with your palms facing down. Bend your knees 90 degrees.

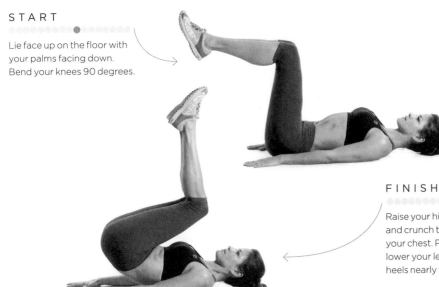

FINISH

Raise your hips off the floor and crunch them towards your chest. Pause, then slowly lower your legs until your heels nearly touch the floor.

147
Abs

Swiss Ball Side Crunch

START

Lie sideways on a Swiss ball and brace your right foot against a wall or a heavy object. Place your fingers behind your ears.

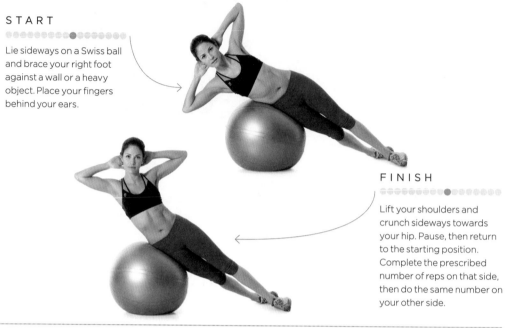

FINISH

Lift your shoulders and crunch sideways towards your hip. Pause, then return to the starting position. Complete the prescribed number of reps on that side, then do the same number on your other side.

Swiss Ball Crunch

START

Lie with your hips, lower back, and shoulders in contact with a Swiss ball and hold a weight plate across your chest

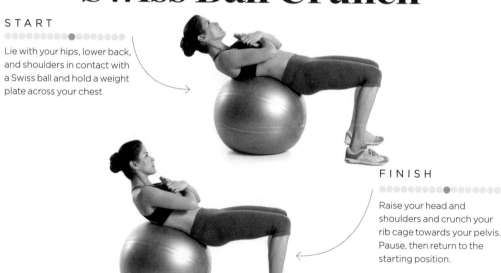

FINISH

Raise your head and shoulders and crunch your rib cage towards your pelvis. Pause, then return to the starting position.

148
Abs

Seated Core Stabilisation

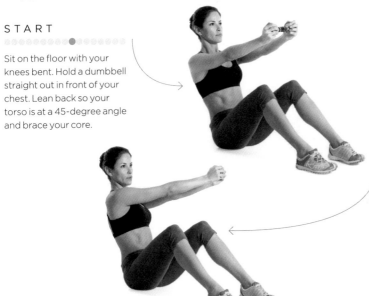

START

Sit on the floor with your knees bent. Hold a dumbbell straight out in front of your chest. Lean back so your torso is at a 45-degree angle and brace your core.

FINISH

Without changing the position of your torso, slowly (take 2 seconds) rotate your arms to the right as far as you can. Pause for 3 seconds. Slowly rotate your arms to the left as far as you can. Pause again, then alternate back and forth for the allotted time.

Slide Out

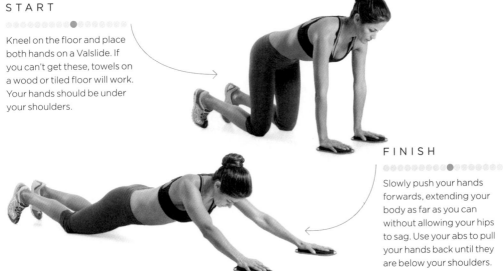

START

Kneel on the floor and place both hands on a Valslide. If you can't get these, towels on a wood or tiled floor will work. Your hands should be under your shoulders.

FINISH

Slowly push your hands forwards, extending your body as far as you can without allowing your hips to sag. Use your abs to pull your hands back until they are below your shoulders.

149
Abs

Plank

Start to get in a press-up position, but bend your elbows and rest your weight on your forearms instead of on your hands. Your body should form a straight line from shoulders to ankles.

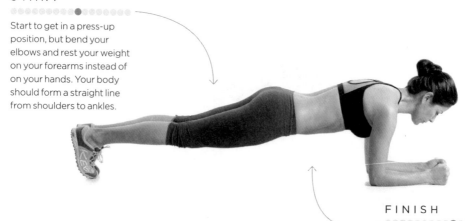

F I N I S H

Brace your core by contracting your abs as if you were about to be punched in the gut. Hold this position as directed.

Side Plank

S T A R T

Lie on your left side with your knees straight. Prop your upper body up on your left elbow and forearm. Brace your core by contracting your abs forcefully.

150
Abs

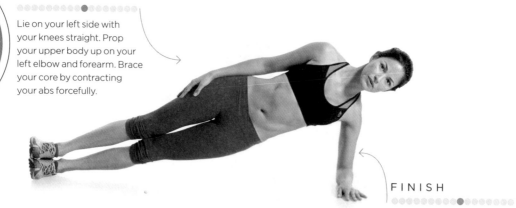

F I N I S H

Raise your hips until your body forms a straight line from your ankles to your shoulders. Hold as directed, then switch sides and repeat.

Hands-Free Side Plank

START

Lie on your left side with your knees straight. Place both of your feet on a bench and cross your arms over your chest. Squeeze your glutes and prop your upper body up on your left shoulder. Brace your core by contracting your abs forcefully.

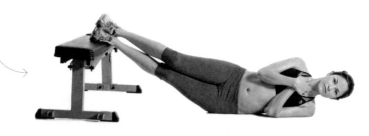

FINISH

Raise your hips until your body forms a straight line from your ankles to your shoulders. Hold for the required duration, then switch sides and repeat.

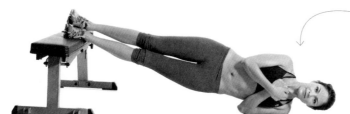

Plank to Press-Up

START

Start to get in a press-up position, but bend your elbows and rest your weight on your forearms instead of on your hands. Your body should form a straight line from your shoulders to your ankles. Brace your core by contracting your abs as if you were about to be punched in the gut.

FINISH

Press your body up into the top position of a press-up by extending your arms one at a time. Pause, then reverse the movement and return to your elbows. That's 1 rep.

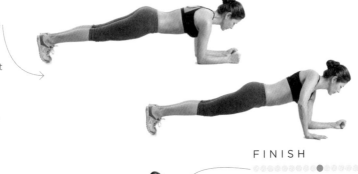

151
Abs

Side Plank and Rotate

START

Lift your body into a side plank, and start with your right arm raised straight above you so that it's perpendicular to the floor

FINISH

Reach under and behind your torso with your right hand, keeping your abs braced. Lift your arm back up to the starting position. That's 1 rep. Do all reps, roll onto your other side, and repeat.

Plank Jumping Jack

START

Start to get in a press-up position, but bend your elbows and rest your weight on your forearms instead of on your hands. Your body should form a straight line from your shoulders to your ankles. Brace your core by contracting your abs as if you were about to be punched in the stomach

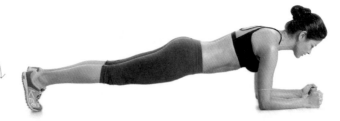

FINISH

Jump your feet out to the sides as if you were performing a jumping jack, making sure that your upper body doesn't rotate. Return your feet to the starting position. That's 1 rep.

Plank and Reach

START

Lower onto all fours and place your weight on your hands so you're in the start position of a press-up. Move your feet so that they're about shoulder-width apart. Your body should form a straight line from your shoulders to your ankles

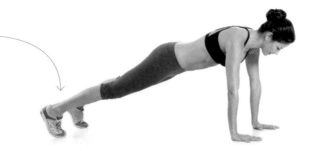

FINISH

Raise your left foot and right arm off the floor and hold. Return to the floor and repeat with your right foot and left arm. That's 1 rep. Make sure that when you raise your arm and leg, your body doesn't rotate and your hips don't rise up.

Plank Frog Tuck

START

Start in a press-up position with your body straight from your shoulders to your ankles

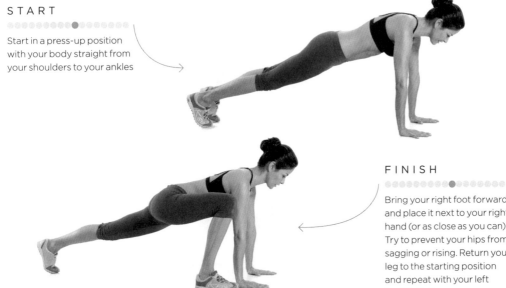

153
Abs

FINISH

Bring your right foot forwards and place it next to your right hand (or as close as you can). Try to prevent your hips from sagging or rising. Return your leg to the starting position and repeat with your left leg. That's 1 rep.

Rolling Plank

START

Begin in the plank position with your body forming a straight line from your shoulders to your ankles. Rotate to your left side and into a side plank.

FINISH

Hold it for 10 seconds, then rotate into a right side plank and hold for another 10 seconds. That's 1 rep. Return to a plank position and repeat.

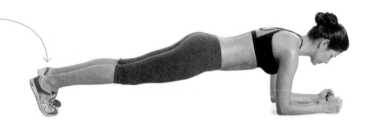

One-Leg Plank

START

Start to get in a press-up position, but bend your elbows and rest your weight on your forearms instead of your hands. Your body should form a straight line from your shoulders to your ankles. Brace your core by contracting your abs as if you were about to be punched in the stomach.

FINISH

Raise one foot a few inches off the floor and hold. Lower your foot and repeat with your other foot. That's 1 rep.

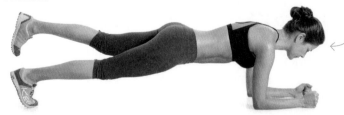

Extended Plank

START

Lower onto all fours and place your weight on your hands so you're in the start position of a press-up. Your body should form a straight line from your shoulders to your ankles

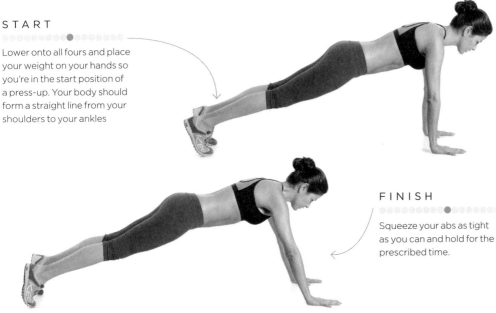

FINISH

Squeeze your abs as tight as you can and hold for the prescribed time.

Side Plank with Row

START

Attach a handle to the low pulley of a cable machine and grab it with your right hand. Brace your core and raise your body into a side plank on your left side.

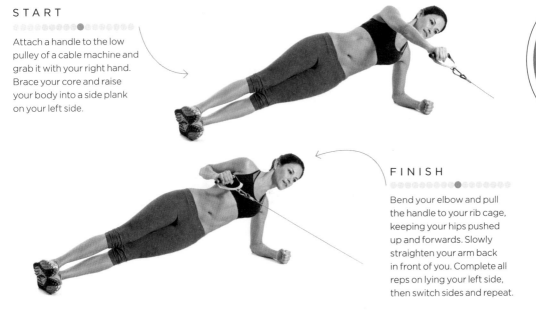

FINISH

Bend your elbow and pull the handle to your rib cage, keeping your hips pushed up and forwards. Slowly straighten your arm back in front of you. Complete all reps on lying your left side, then switch sides and repeat.

155
Abs

Front Plank with Pulldown

START

Attach a handle to the high pulley of a cable machine and grab it in your right hand. Start to get in a press-up position, but bend your elbows and rest your weight on your left forearm and feet. Your body should form a straight line from your shoulders to your ankles.

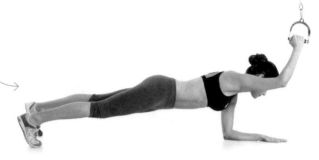

FINISH

With your palm facing your body, bend your right elbow and pull the cable down towards the floor, and then return to the starting position. Complete all reps, switch arms, and repeat

---

Mountain Climber

START

Assume a press-up position with your arms completely straight. Your body should form a straight line from your shoulders to your ankles.

156
Abs

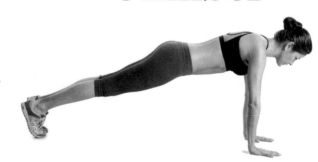

FINISH

Lift your right foot off the floor and slowly raise your knee as close to your chest as you can. Return to the starting position and repeat with your left leg. Continue alternating for the prescribed number of reps or time

Ball Mountain Climber

START

Place your hands on a Swiss ball and assume a press-up position with your arms completely straight. Your body should form a straight line from your shoulders to your ankles.

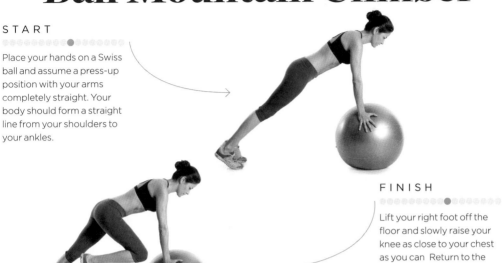

FINISH

Lift your right foot off the floor and slowly raise your knee as close to your chest as you can Return to the starting position and repeat with your left leg. Continue alternating for the prescribed number of reps or time.

Cross-Body Climber

START

Assume a press-up position with your arms completely straight. Your body should form a straight line from your shoulders to your ankles.

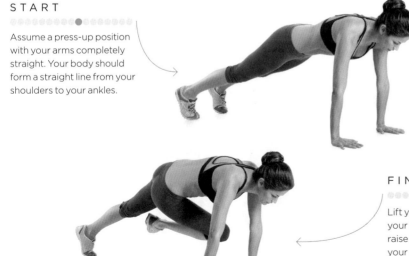

FINISH

Lift your right knee towards your left elbow, lower, then raise your left knee toward your right elbow. That's 1 rep.

157
Abs

Dumbbell Reverse Chops

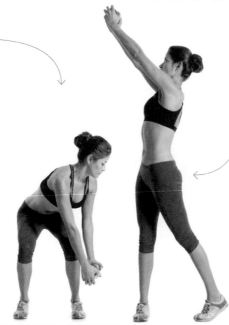

START

Stand with your feet shoulder-width apart. Grab a dumbbell and hold it with both hands just outside your left ankle. Brace your core.

FINISH

In one movement pull the dumbbell up past your right shoulder as you rotate your torso to the right. Reverse the movement to return to the starting position. Complete the prescribed number of reps on one side, then do the same number starting with the dumbbell outside your right ankle, rotating to your left.

Band Tight Rotation

START

Attach a resistance band to a stable object at waist height. Clasp the band with both hands and stand so that your right side faces the anchor, holding the band in front of your chest. Step away until you feel light tension.

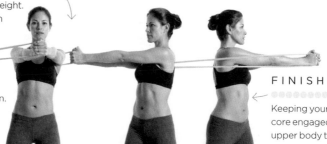

FINISH

Keeping your hips square and core engaged, rotate your upper body to the right so your arms are in line with your right shoulder. That's 1 rep. Reverse, quickly twisting all the way back the other way. Continue alternating quickly for the prescribed number of reps. On the next set, stand with your right side facing the anchor.

Low Cable Chop

START

Attach a rope handle to the low pulley of a cable station. Stand tall with your feet shoulder-width apart, your knees slightly bent, and grab the rope with both hands at arm's length in front of your left hip

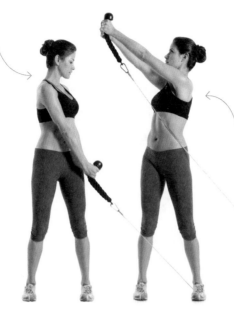

FINISH

Brace your core, and in one movement pull the rope past your right shoulder as you simultaneously rotate your torso to the right. Reverse the movement to return to the starting position. Complete the prescribed number of reps to your right, then do the same number rotating left.

Cable Core Press

START

Attach a handle to a cable machine at chest height. Grab the handle with your hands clasped and stand with your right side facing the weight stack. Spread your feet about shoulder-width apart.

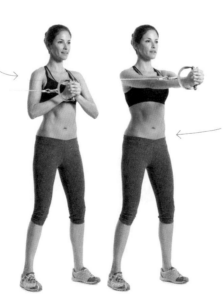

FINISH

Step away from the stack until you feel tension in the cable. Hold the handle against your chest and slowly press your arms in front of you until they're completely straight. Hold for 2 seconds, then return your hands to the starting position. Do all your reps, then turn around and repeat with your left side facing the weight stack.

159
Abs

Swiss Ball Rollout

START

Sit on your knees in front of a Swiss ball, and place your forearms and fist on the ball. Your elbows should be bent about 90 degrees.

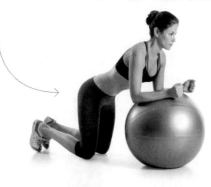

FINISH

Keeping your core braced, slowly roll the ball forward, straightening your arms and extending your body as far as you can without allowing your lower back to collapse. Use your abs to pull the ball back to your knees.

Swiss Ball Stir-The-Pot

160
Abs

START

Assume a plank position with your forearms on a Swiss ball. Your body should form a straight line from your shoulders to your ankles. Squeeze your abs and glutes as hard as you can.

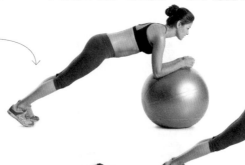

FINISH

Use your forearms to move the ball in small circles while keeping the rest of your body in the original position. Make one circle moving to the right and then one to the left. That's 1 rep.

Swiss Ball Pike

START

Assume a press-up position with your arms completely straight. Position your hands slightly wider than, and in line with, your shoulders. Rest your shins on a Swiss ball. Your body should form a straight line from your shoulders to your ankles

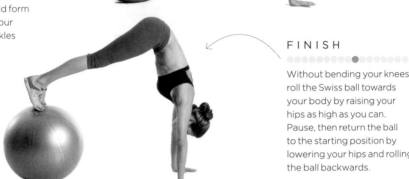

FINISH

Without bending your knees, roll the Swiss ball towards your body by raising your hips as high as you can. Pause, then return the ball to the starting position by lowering your hips and rolling the ball backwards.

Swiss Ball Jackknife

START

Assume a press-up position with your arms completely straight. Rest your shins on a Swiss ball so that your body forms a straight line from your shoulders to your ankles.

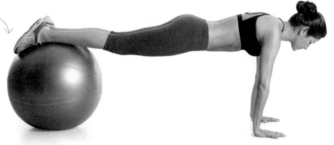

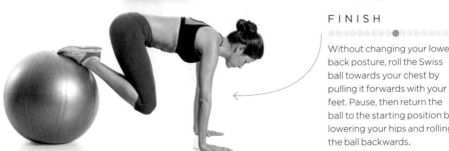

FINISH

Without changing your lower back posture, roll the Swiss ball towards your chest by pulling it forwards with your feet. Pause, then return the ball to the starting position by lowering your hips and rolling the ball backwards.

161
Abs

Medicine Ball Twist

START

Sit on the floor with your knees bent and your feet flat. Hold a medicine ball, with your arms straight out in front of your chest. Lean back so your torso is at a 45-degree angle to the floor.

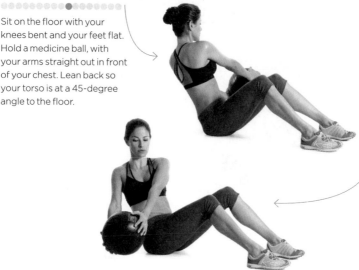

FINISH

Brace your core and rotate to the right as far as you can. Pause, then reverse your movement and twist all the way back to the left as far as you can.

Medicine Ball Side Slam

START

Grab a medicine ball and hold it above your head. Your arms should be slightly bent and your feet shoulder-width apart. Brace your abs.

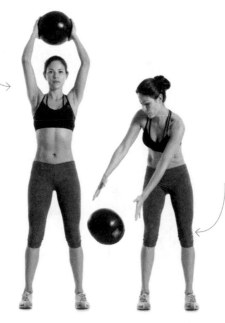

FINISH

Forcefully slam the ball towards the outside of your right foot as hard as you can. Pick the ball up and repeat, this time slamming toward the outside of your left foot. That's 1 rep

162
Abs

Medicine Ball Rotation

START

Grab a medicine ball and stand sideways about 1m (3ft) from a brick or concrete wall, with your left side facing the wall. Hold the ball at chest level with your arms straight and rotate your torso to your right.

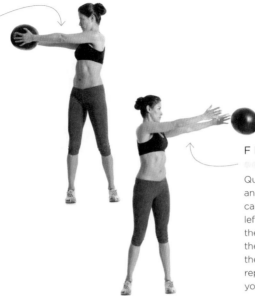

FINISH

Quickly switch directions and throw as hard as you can against the wall to your left. As the ball rebounds off the wall, catch it and repeat the movement. Complete the prescribed number of repetitions, then repeat with your right side facing the wall.

Medicine Ball Slam

START

Grab a medicine ball and hold it above your head. Your arms should be slightly bent and your feet roughly shoulder-width apart.

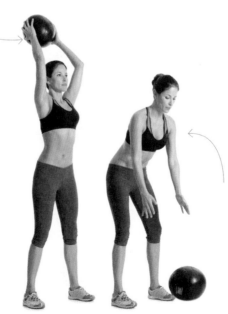

FINISH

Forcefully slam the ball to the floor in front of you as hard as you can. Pick the ball up and repeat the move.

163
Abs

Dumbbell Side Bend

START

Stand with your feet shoulder-width apart. Hold a dumbbell in your right hand at your side with your arms straight.

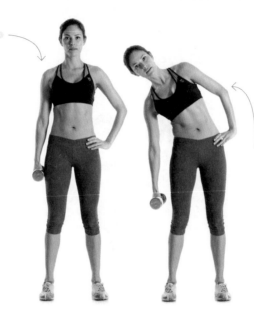

FINISH

Squeeze your abs tight and, without twisting your upper body, slowly bend to the right as far as you can, lowering the weight towards your right knee. Pause, then slowly return to an upright position. Complete all reps to the right, hold the dumbbell in your left hand, and repeat on your other side.

Dead Bug

START

Lie face up on the floor with your arms at your sides. Raise your legs off the floor so that your hips and knees are bent 90 degrees.

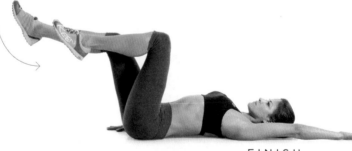

FINISH

Brace your abs. Bring your left knee towards your chest a few inches and your right knee away from your chest. Raise your left hand up and over your head. Now switch legs as you raise your right arm overhead and lower your left arm back. That's 1 rep.

164
Abs

Side Pillar Jack

START

Lie on your left side with your knees straight. Prop your upper body up on your left elbow and forearm. Raise your hips until your body forms a straight line from your shoulders to your ankles

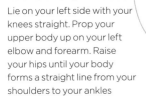
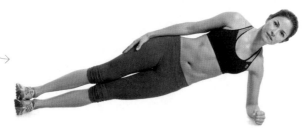

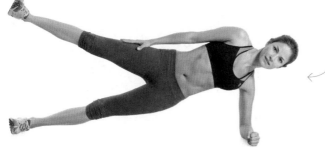

FINISH

Raise your top leg as high as you can and hold it that way for 2 seconds. Lower it back to the starting position. That's 1 rep. Perform the prescribed number of reps, then turn around so that you're lying on your right side and repeat

Around The World

START

Place both feet on a bench and assume a press-up position. Your body should form a straight line from your shoulders to your ankles.

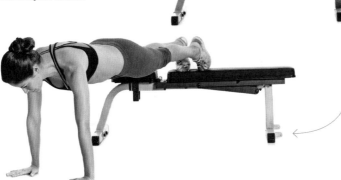

FINISH

Brace your core and, without dropping your hips or moving your feet, make a full revolution around the bench by "walking" your hands all the way around it. That's 1 rep.

165 Abs

PART THREE

COMPLETE WORKOUT PLANNER

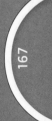

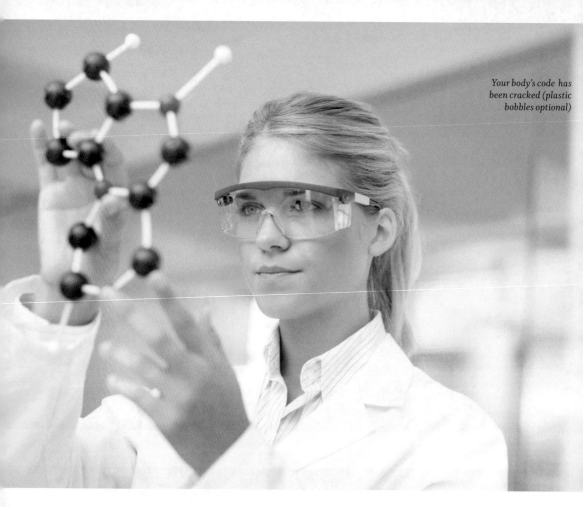

Workout science

*Before picking one of the 12 workouts that follow, or creating your own, ensure you get
the most out of your gym time by brushing up on a little biology and physics*

When you visit the gym, you
probably make your way into
one of two areas: the cardio
machines or spinning class.
Both offer stress relief, burn calories and will
improve your overall health. And while we'd
never suggest that you completely ignore an
activity you enjoy, using either of these
methods is not the best way to see rapid
results – especially when your biggest

challenge is simply finding time. You need an
exercise plan that guarantees every second of
your gym time will result in a flatter tummy.
That's why we created *Flat Belly Workouts*. It
doesn't matter if you've been exercising for
10 years or never set foot in the gym – you've
never experienced workouts like this before.

Each workout you'll find in this section has
a different focus, whether that's legs, arms,
top-half or total body. However, they all have

one thing in common: they will all burn fat and uncover your abs. That's because they all have a combination of exercises to tone all your muscles and innovative movements that challenge your core and keep your workouts fun and engaging. None of them require you do them more than three days a week, but they will exhaustively work all of your muscles, so you'll need rest days to ensure you keep operating at peak efficiency.

THE FALL OF MACHINES

These workouts offer everything you'll ever need to transform your body as efficiently as possible. But as you flick through and check them out, you might notice something: there are hardly any machines. That's not a mistake. If you want some insight into why so many people struggle to lose weight, just step into any gym. There, in that big space, you have a template for obesity: lots of cardio equipment lined up in front of televisions. Rows and rows of beautiful exercise machines, strategically organised to help you work all your muscles.

The gym owners aren't stupid. They built these facilities to make you feel at home and comfortable. Machines are welcoming, convenient, and enjoyable. But there's nothing worse than spending hundreds of pounds on a membership, hours and hours in a gym and still not seeing the results that you're after. While there might be several reasons for this, the machines deserve at least some of the blame. After all, machines – for all their convenience – are less effective at making changes to your body.

In fact, both dumbbells and bodyweight resistance are better alternatives and can help you burn more calories, say researchers from Columbia University. They found that free weights activate more muscle fibres, which results in more calories burned. While you won't notice a difference, your body will. That's because the non-mechanical approach allows you to perform your entire workout in fewer exercises. Think about it: machines target each body part specifically, whereas it's much more efficient to do exercises that work multiple muscles. So instead of doing leg curls, leg extensions and the thigh machine, you could just do lunges – and see better results in a fraction of the time.

Faster results are one thing, but aren't machines safer? After all, you're much more likely to drop a dumbbell than experience a machine falling apart. However, many machines are more likely to cause injury than free weights because they focus on one muscle group without strengthening the others around it. If you don't strengthen supporting groups eventually muscles get pulled, sprained or torn. That's why our plans remove most machines from the equation and, at times, remove all equipment so you can do your entire workout at home. Your bodyweight can help you score the ultimate body.

> **Instead of using leg machines just do lunges – you'll see better results in a fraction of the time**

The machine-free approach will help you bust out of a slump and put you on the fast track to shrinking your belly.

YOUR ABS – REVEALED

By now you might feel that you have a pretty good idea of what exactly what it takes to flip the switch on the ultimate body makeover and get toned muscle and a flat belly. So let's try a little quiz.

Which of the following is true:
  A **Abs are the key to a flatter belly**
  B **Gimmick devices and supplements will help eliminate your muffin top.**
  C **Crunches are the best exercise for your core**

Turn the page…

169
Science

So what did you pick? Hopefully you were waiting for (d) None of the above. You see, the lessons of the lean are not what they used to be, which means the methods of changing your body are not what you commonly see in the gym. So let's start with the basics: the terms core and abs are not interchangeable. Crunches work your abs. But for the biggest benefits, you need to work your entire core, which is made up of no less than nine distinct

Crunches work 64% of your six-pack. Planks work 100%

muscle groups, outlined in the diagram opposite. Together they help to stabilise your entire body.

That's the real purpose of your core: to prevent movement. So when you are doing crunches – or creating movement – you're doing the opposite of what was intended for your body. While crunches feel like they're doing something, they're actually one of the last exercises you want to include in an ab-revealing routine. Not only do they put your back at risk for injury, they also work your muscles less than the alternatives. In fact, a study published in the *Journal of Strength and Conditioning Research* found that crunches create a 64 percent activation of your six-pack muscles. That sounds great until you realize that Canadian researchers found that a variation of the basic plank achieves 100 percent activation of the same muscles.

The message is clear, the more you train your abs for stability – with planks, side planks etc – the better you'll look. The best part: you'll barely have to move, which should eliminate your strains and pains. Just beware. The exercises in this programme may look easy but they will challenge you like never before. We're confident there is no faster route to a flat belly.

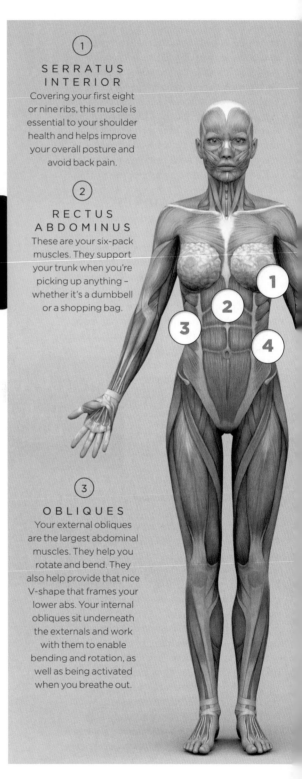

1

SERRATUS INTERIOR
Covering your first eight or nine ribs, this muscle is essential to your shoulder health and helps improve your overall posture and avoid back pain.

2

RECTUS ABDOMINUS
These are your six-pack muscles. They support your trunk when you're picking up anything – whether it's a dumbbell or a shopping bag.

3

OBLIQUES
Your external obliques are the largest abdominal muscles. They help you rotate and bend. They also help provide that nice V-shape that frames your lower abs. Your internal obliques sit underneath the externals and work with them to enable bending and rotation, as well as being activated when you breathe out.

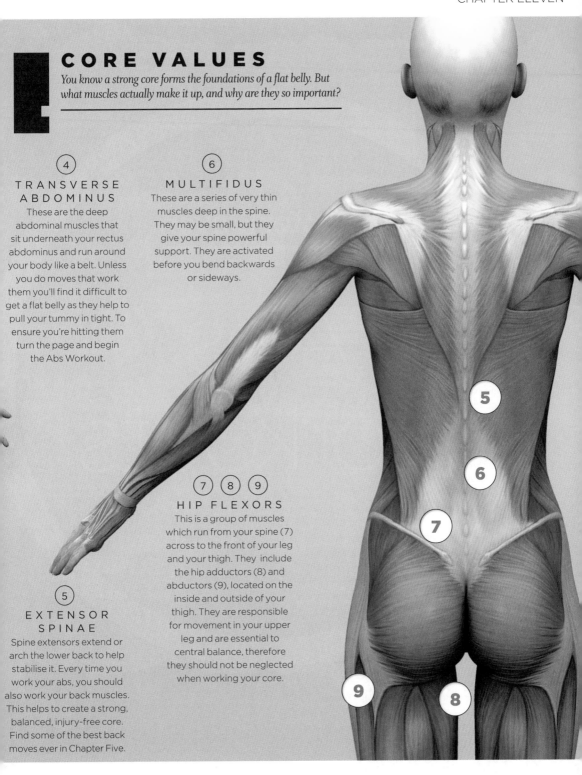

CORE VALUES

You know a strong core forms the foundations of a flat belly. But what muscles actually make it up, and why are they so important?

(4)

TRANSVERSE ABDOMINUS

These are the deep abdominal muscles that sit underneath your rectus abdominus and run around your body like a belt. Unless you do moves that work them you'll find it difficult to get a flat belly as they help to pull your tummy in tight. To ensure you're hitting them turn the page and begin the Abs Workout.

(6)

MULTIFIDUS

These are a series of very thin muscles deep in the spine. They may be small, but they give your spine powerful support. They are activated before you bend backwards or sideways.

(7) (8) (9)

HIP FLEXORS

This is a group of muscles which run from your spine (7) across to the front of your leg and your thigh. They include the hip adductors (8) and abductors (9), located on the inside and outside of your thigh. They are responsible for movement in your upper leg and are essential to central balance, therefore they should not be neglected when working your core.

(5)

EXTENSOR SPINAE

Spine extensors extend or arch the lower back to help stabilise it. Every time you work your abs, you should also work your back muscles. This helps to create a strong, balanced, injury-free core. Find some of the best back moves ever in Chapter Five.

Abs workouts

INTENSE, TOTAL-BODY WORKOUTS
FOR A FLAT-BELLY, FAST

The three programmes in this chapter are the most abs-specific. Of course, you'll still get a flat belly from any of the plans in this book, these are simply the ones that focus most closely on your core: they consist of the Abs Workout that follows, plus the Fastest Workout Ever (p182) and the Bodyweight Abs Workout (p184) (now never have an excuse to miss a session again).

In order to keep getting results at the same rate you need to change your workout every 4-6 weeks. This is because your body will grow accustomed to the challenge and your gains will plateau. So once you've completed four weeks of the Abs Workout, pick another from this chapter, or the next, and use that. Then switch again after another four weeks. It's a good idea to keep three or four different workouts in rotation.

BEFORE YOU BEGIN

Start each workout with a five-minute warm-up. A circuit of bodyweight moves, as you'll find in the Bodyweight Abs Workout (p184), works well, or you can hop on the treadmill. Your heart rate should be elevated, and you should have light perspiration before you begin.

WHAT YOU NEED

The workouts in this chapter only simple equipment (or none at all) so you can do them at home. Or, if you prefer, head to the gym. Start with lighter weights to assess your comfort level, then increase the weight as your strength increases. If you are using a challenging enough weight you should be finding the final sets of each exercise hard and you might not complete all the reps. This is good, as it shows you are pushing your muscles to the limit. If you can't complete all the reps in the first set, however, the weight you are using is too heavy so go lighter

next time. As you progress you'll become stronger so you should up the weights. The workout charts will help you keep track. Remember, don't be afraid that using bigger weights will make you bulky. It won't. That happens to men because they have higher levels of muscle-building testosterone. As a woman you will become more toned. This new lean muscle will melt more fat as it requires more calories for your body to maintain. This will allow you to eat the type of foods you enjoy without feeling guilty.

STEPPING IT UP

All you need is three days a week of exercise and you'll completely transform the way you look. However, if you want to do additional activity, such as cardio, perform it on the days you're not schedule to work out. For instance, if you exercise Monday, Wednesday, and Friday, you could do cardio

> All you need is three days a week of exercise and you'll completely transform the way you look

on Tuesday and Thursday. In fact, many people find having something scheduled every weekday is a good way to get into the habit of exercising regularly. Just make sure you give yourself at least one full day off every week. Weekend days normally work best for this if you work Monday to Friday.

READY TO START

Turn the page for the first plan which consists of two parts. Alternate between Workout A and Workout B three days a week, resting for at least a day between each session. So if you plan to exercise Monday, Wednesday, and Friday, you'd do Workout A on Monday, Workout B on Wednesday, and Workout A again on Friday. The next week, you'd do Workout B on Monday and Friday, and Workout A on Wednesday.

173
Abs workouts

Abs Workout A

30-40 minutes

Welcome to the first stage of your new body. Use this in conjunction with Abs Workout B, starting on page 178, for your complete tummy-toning plan

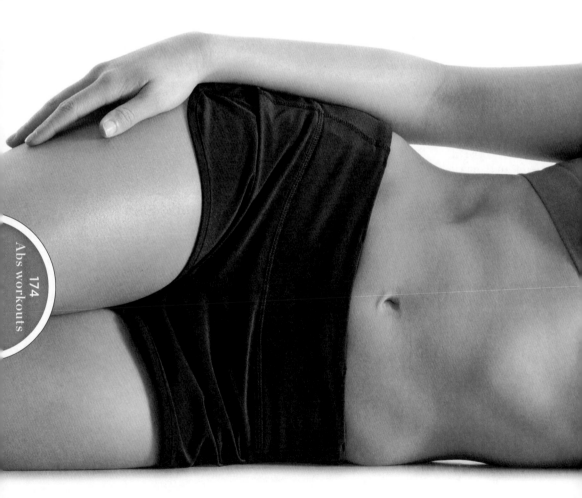

HOW TO DO IT

● Each workout consists of four circuits. Perform the exercises in each circuit in the order shown, aiming for the number of reps specified. Do 1 set of each in turn, rest for 2 minutes, then go back to the first exercise in the circuit and repeat until you've completed all the sets. Then move on to the next circuit. As you complete each set, fill in the number of reps you do in the space provided. It will help you keep track of your progress and will also be a powerful motivator.

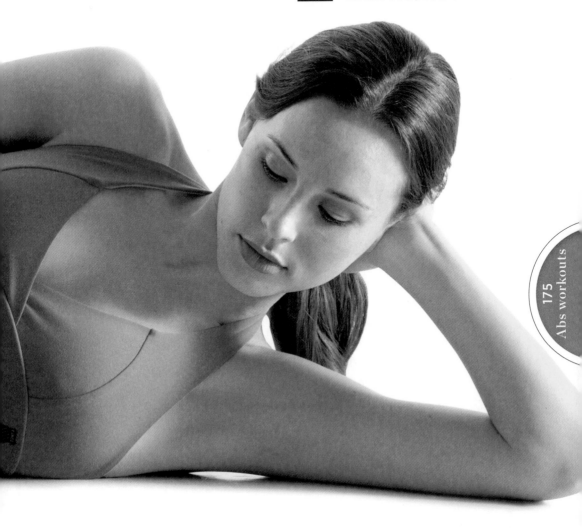

175

Abs workouts

Women'sHealth

Abs Workout A: Circuits A-B

CIRCUIT A

Exercise		WEEK 1		WEEK 2		WEEK 3		WEEK 4	
		Weight	Reps	Weight	Reps	Weight	Reps	Weight	Reps
Swiss Ball Chest Press, p90 (3 sets, 12 reps/side)	DAY 1								
	DAY 2								
Swissball Jackknife, p161 (3 sets, 10 reps)	DAY 1								
	DAY 2								
One-arm Row, p96 (3 sets, 15 reps/side)	DAY 1								
	DAY 2								

CIRCUIT B

Exercise		WEEK 1		WEEK 2		WEEK 3		WEEK 4	
		Weight	Reps	Weight	Reps	Weight	Reps	Weight	Reps
Squat Thrusts, p112 (3 sets, 10-15 reps)	DAY 1								
	DAY 2								
Dumbbell Deadlift, p141 (3 sets, 12 reps/side)	DAY 1								
	DAY 2								
Jump Lunges, p135 (3 sets, 20 reps)	DAY 1								
	DAY 2								

USE THESE CHARTS TO KEEP TRACK OF YOUR PROGRESS. TRY TO INCREASE WEIGHTS AS SOON AS YOU FEEL ABLE. FOR A FULL WORKOUT DESCRIPTION SEE THE BEGINNING OF THIS CHAPTER AND FOR FULL DETAILS OF THE MOVES TURN TO

Women'sHealth — Abs Workout A: Circuits C-D

CIRCUIT C

		WEEK 1		WEEK 2		WEEK 3		WEEK 4	
		Weight	Reps	Weight	Reps	Weight	Reps	Weight	Reps
Pullover, p102 (3 sets, 10-12 reps)	DAY 1								
	DAY 2								
Overhead Extensions, p101 (3 sets, 6-10 reps)	DAY 1								
	DAY 2								
Single-leg Squat, p132 (3 sets, 10 reps/side)	DAY 1								
	DAY 2								

CIRCUIT D

		WEEK 1		WEEK 2		WEEK 3		WEEK 2	
		Weight	Reps	Weight	Reps	Weight	Reps	Weight	Reps
Dumbbell Push Press, p114 (3 sets, 10-12 reps)	DAY 1								
	DAY 2								
Swissball Stir-The-Pot, p160 (3 sets, 60 sec)	DAY 1								
	DAY 2								
Bodyweight Squat, p127 (3 sets, 10-15 reps)	DAY 1								
	DAY 2								

Abs Workout B

30-40 minutes

Perform this workout alternately with Abs Workout A, which begins on page 174, three days a week, so you never perform the same workout sequentially

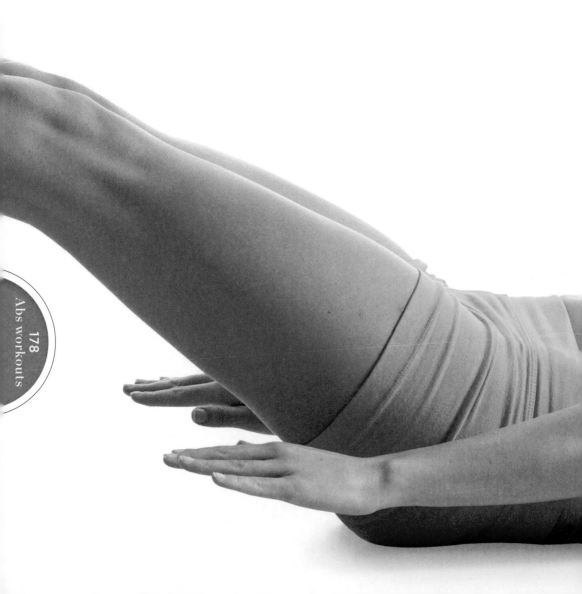

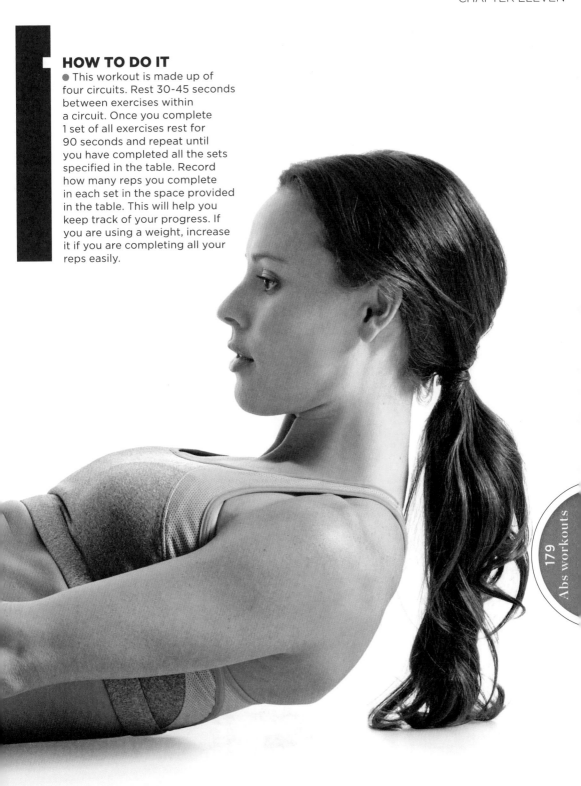

HOW TO DO IT

● This workout is made up of four circuits. Rest 30-45 seconds between exercises within a circuit. Once you complete 1 set of all exercises rest for 90 seconds and repeat until you have completed all the sets specified in the table. Record how many reps you complete in each set in the space provided in the table. This will help you keep track of your progress. If you are using a weight, increase it if you are completing all your reps easily.

Abs Workout B: Circuits A-B

CIRCUIT A

		WEEK 1		WEEK 2		WEEK 3		WEEK 4	
		Weight	Reps	Weight	Reps	Weight	Reps	Weight	Reps
Lunge, p130 (2 sets, 10 reps/side)	DAY 1								
	DAY 2								
Mountain Climbers, p156 (2 sets, 20 reps)	DAY 1		Reps		Reps		Reps		Reps
	DAY 2		Reps		Reps		Reps		Reps
Swissball Rollout, p160 (3 sets, 15 reps)	DAY 1		Reps		Reps		Reps		Reps
	DAY 2		Reps		Reps		Reps		Reps
Swissball Jackknife, p161 (2 sets, 8-10 reps)	DAY 1		Reps		Reps		Reps		Reps
	DAY 2		Reps		Reps		Reps		Reps
Lateral Raise, p106 (2 sets, 10 reps)	DAY 1	Weight	Reps	Weight	Reps	Weight	Reps	Weight	Reps
	DAY 2	Weight	Reps	Weight	Reps	Weight	Reps	Weight	Reps

CIRCUIT B

		WEEK 1		WEEK 2		WEEK 3		WEEK 4	
		Weight	Reps	Weight	Reps	Weight	Reps	Weight	Reps
Lunge to Curl to Press, p124 (4 sets, 6 per leg)	DAY 1	Weight	Reps	Weight	Reps	Weight	Reps	Weight	Reps
	DAY 2	Weight	Reps	Weight	Reps	Weight	Reps	Weight	Reps

USE THESE CHARTS TO KEEP TRACK OF YOUR PROGRESS. TRY TO INCREASE WEIGHTS AS SOON AS YOU FEEL ABLE. FOR A FULL WORKOUT DESCRIPTION SEE THE BEGINNING OF THIS CHAPTER AND FOR DETAILS OF THE MOVES TURN TO THE PAGES INDICATED. YOU CAN CONTINUE THIS WORKOUT BEYOND FOUR WEEKS, PROGRESSING AS YOU FEEL ABLE, OR SWAP FOR ANOTHER

Women'sHealth | Abs Workout B: Circuits C-D

CIRCUIT C

Exercise		WEEK 1		WEEK 2		WEEK 3		WEEK 4	
Negative Chin-up, p99 (4 sets, 10 reps)	DAY1		Reps		Reps		Reps		Reps
	DAY2		Reps		Reps		Reps		Reps
Dumbbell Deadlift, p141 (4 sets, 15 reps)	DAY1	Weight	Reps	Weight	Reps	Weight	Reps	Weight	Reps
	DAY2		Weight		Weight		Weight		Weight
Squat Jump, p129 (4 sets, 30sec)	DAY1		Reps		Reps		Reps		Reps
	DAY2		Reps		Reps		Reps		Reps
Rolling Plank, p154 (4 sets, 45sec)	DAY1		Reps		Reps		Reps		Reps
	DAY2		Reps		Reps		Reps		Reps

CIRCUIT D

Exercise		WEEK 1		WEEK 2		WEEK 3		WEEK 4	
Swiss Ball Chest Press, p90 (3 sets, 10-12 reps)	DAY1	Weight	Reps	Weight	Reps	Weight	Reps	Weight	Reps
	DAY2	Weight	Reps	Weight	Reps	Weight	Reps	Weight	Reps
Step-up and Press, p124 (3 sets, 15 reps/side)	DAY1	Weight	Reps	Weight	Reps	Weight	Reps	Weight	Reps
	DAY2		Weight	Reps	Weight	Reps	Weight	Reps	Weight	Reps
Lunge and One-Arm Press, p116 (3 sets, 8 reps/side)	DAY1	Weight	Reps	Weight	Reps	Weight	Reps	Weight	Reps
	DAY2		Weight	Reps	Weight	Reps	Weight	Reps	Weight	Reps

181
Abs workouts

Fastest Workout Ever Created

10 minutes

This workout takes you out of your normal comfort zone and into the fat-burning one. And it's so simple it'll appear almost too good to be true. But it's been proven to challenge any woman – from beginners to experts – and is the fastest way to blast stubborn ab flab.

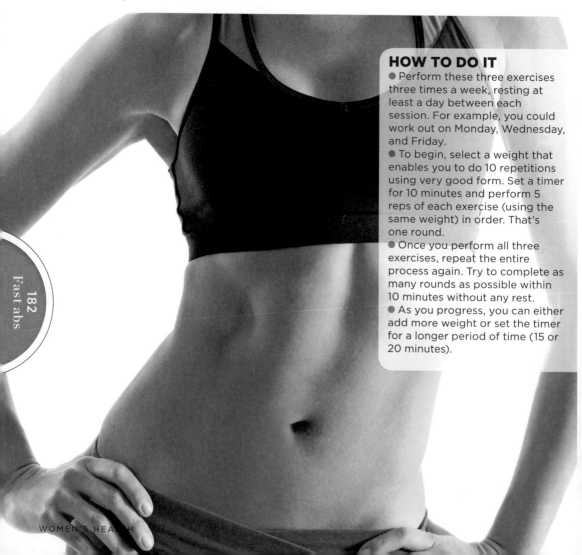

HOW TO DO IT

● Perform these three exercises three times a week, resting at least a day between each session. For example, you could work out on Monday, Wednesday, and Friday.

● To begin, select a weight that enables you to do 10 repetitions using very good form. Set a timer for 10 minutes and perform 5 reps of each exercise (using the same weight) in order. That's one round.

● Once you perform all three exercises, repeat the entire process again. Try to complete as many rounds as possible within 10 minutes without any rest.

● As you progress, you can either add more weight or set the timer for a longer period of time (15 or 20 minutes).

Women'sHealth

The Fastest Workout Ever

		WEEK 1		WEEK 2		WEEK 3		WEEK 4	
		Weight	Rounds completed	Weight	Rounds completed	Weight	Rounds completed	Weight	Rounds completed
Goblet Squat to Press, p113 (10 reps per round)	MON		Rounds completed		Rounds completed		Rounds completed		Rounds completed
	WED	Weight	Rounds completed	Weight	Rounds completed	Weight	Rounds completed	Weight	Rounds completed
	FRI	Weight	Rounds completed	Weight	Rounds completed	Weight	Rounds completed	Weight	Rounds completed
Inverted Row, p93 (10 reps per round)	MON		Rounds completed		Rounds completed		Rounds completed		Rounds completed
	WED		Rounds completed		Rounds completed		Rounds completed		Rounds completed
	FRI		Rounds completed		Rounds completed		Rounds completed		Rounds completed
Step-up and Press, p124 (10 reps per round)	MON	Weight	Rounds completed	Weight	Rounds completed	Weight	Rounds completed	Weight	Rounds completed
	WED	Weight	Rounds completed	Weight	Rounds completed	Weight	Rounds completed	Weight	Rounds completed
	FRI	Weight	Rounds completed	Weight	Rounds completed	Weight	Rounds completed	Weight	Rounds completed

183
Fast abs

FLAT BELLY WORKOUTS

Bodyweight Abs Workouts

45 minutes

Dumbbells and barbells are great, but you can outsmart fat and blast cellulite using just your bodyweight. This versatile workout requires only one piece of equipment: you. The movements require you utilize your entire body and balance several muscles at the same time, so they'll not only increase the intensity of your workout, but also fire up your metabolism.

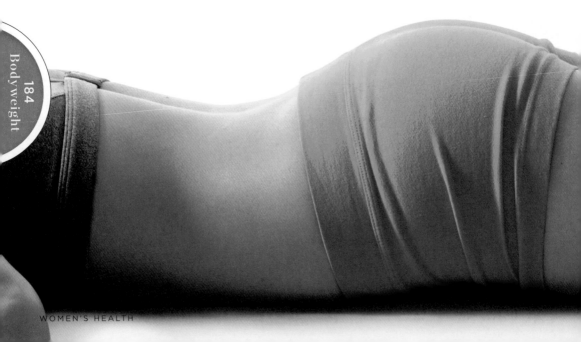

HOW TO DO IT

- Do one of the folllowing workouts 3 days a week. Rest a day between each session. So you might lift weights on Monday, Wednesday and Friday.
- Each workout consists of four phases: a dynamic warm-up, bodyweight exercises, core movements and then a cool down. Perform all of the exercises as straight sets. That is, do all of the required sets and reps of an exercise before moving on to the next.
- Rest for 30 seconds after each set during the warm-up and core work, and 60 seconds between the bodyweight sets.
- Change which phase you do each week. Work up to Phase 4, then mix and match to you keep your body guessing.

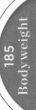

185
Bodyweight

Women'sHealth

Bodyweight Abs Phase One

	WEEK 1			WEEK 2			WEEK 3			WEEK 4		
	MON	WED	FRI	MON	WED	FRI	MON	WED	FRI	MON	WED	FRI

WARM UP

Inchworms, p122
1 set, 10 reps

Lunge and Reach, p118
1 set, 5 reps/leg

Squat to stand, p112
1 set, 10 reps

BODYWEIGHT

Press-ups, p83
3 sets, 8-12 reps

Inverted Row, p93
3 sets, 8-12 reps

Bodyweight Squat, p142 3 sets, 10 reps

Hip raise, p116
3 sets, 10 reps

CORE

Around the World,
p165 2 sets, 1 rep

Cross-Body Climbers, p157
4 sets, 25-30 reps

COOLDOWNS

Light jog and stretch

Women'sHealth
Bodyweight Abs Phase Two

		WEEK 1			WEEK 2			WEEK 3			WEEK 4		
		MON	WED	FRI	MON	WED	FRI	MON	WED	FRI	MON	WED	FRI
WARM UP													
Jumping jack, p111 — 1 set, 20 reps													
Inchworms & Press-ups, p122 & 83, 1 set, 5 reps													
Lunge and reach, p118 — 1 set, 20 reps													
BODYWEIGHT													
Press-ups, p83 — 3 sets, 12-15 reps	Set 1												
	Set 2												
	Set 3												
Inverted Row, p93 — 3 sets, 12-15 reps	Set 1												
	Set 2												
	Set 3												
Hip Raise, p142 — 3 sets, 12 reps	Set 1												
	Set 2												
	Set 3												
CORE													
Around the Worlds, p165 2 sets, 1 rep	Set 1												
	Set 2												
Cross-Body Climbers, p157 — 4 sets, 25-30 reps	Set 1												
	Set 2												
	Set 3												
	Set 4												
COOLDOWNS													
Light jog and stretch													

187
Bodyweight

Women's Health

Bodyweight Abs Phase Three

		WEEK 1			WEEK 2			WEEK 3			WEEK 4		
		MON	WED	FRI	MON	WED	FRI	MON	WED	FRI	MON	WED	FRI
WARM UP													
Press-ups, p83 — 1 set, 15 reps													
Inchworms, p122 — 1 set, 15 reps													
Lunge and Reach, p118 — 1 set, 6 reps each side													
Squat to stand, p112 — 1 set, 12 reps													
BODYWEIGHT													
Press-ups, p83 — 4 sets, 8-12 reps	Set 1												
	Set 2												
	Set 3												
	Set 4												
Inverted Row, p93 — 4 sets, 10-15 reps	Set 1												
	Set 2												
	Set 3												
	Set 4												
Hip raise, p142 — 4 sets, 10 reps	Set 1												
	Set 2												
	Set 3												
	Set 4												
CORE													
Around the worlds, p165 — 4 sets, 1 rep	Set 1												
	Set 2												
	Set 3												
	Set 4												
Cross-Boy Climbers, p157 — 4 sets, 10-15 reps	Set 1												
	Set 2												
	Set 3												
	Set 4												
COOLDOWNS													
Light jog and stretch													

Women'sHealth — *Bodyweight Abs Phase Four*

		WEEK 1			WEEK 2			WEEK 3			WEEK 4	
		MON	WED	FRI	MON	WED	FRI	MON	WED	FRI	MON	WED	FRI
WARM UP													
Jumping jack, p111 — 1 set, 20 reps													
Inchworms & Press-ups, p122 & 83 1 set, 8 reps													
Lunge and reach, p118 — 1 set, 6 per side													
BODYWEIGHT													
Press-ups, p83 — 4 sets, 12–15 per side	Set 1												
	Set 2												
	Set 3												
	Set 4												
Inverted Row, p93 — 4 sets, 15–20 per side	Set 1												
	Set 2												
	Set 3												
	Set 4												
Hip raise, p142 — 4 sets, Reps 12–15	Set 1												
	Set 2												
	Set 3												
	Set 4												
CORE													
Around the World, p165 — 4 sets, 2 reps	Set 1												
	Set 2												
	Set 3												
	Set 4												
Cross Body Climbers, p1 — 4 sets, 25–30 reps	Set 1												
	Set 2												
	Set 3												
	Set 4												
COOLDOWNS													
Light jog and stretch													

189
Bodyweight

Chapter Twelve

Smart workouts

FOUR CHALLENGING NEW
WORKOUTS TAILOR-MADE
TO YOUR TARGETS

Just as you have good and bad diets, the same could be said about your gym routine. That's why we got some of the world's best experts to design workouts using the moves described in this book, that will help you reach your targets, fast. Each one is designed to keep you working hard and ensure you keep seeing results.

So, once you've completed the Abs Workouts in the previous chapter turn here to really start honing your body. Whether you want to get ready for the beach or fit into your favourite pair of jeans, anything is possible. All you need to do is follow the plans and work hard. The results will follow.

But here's the key: don't change the exercises unless noted by the experts. These workouts were specifically designed to help you get in the best shape of your life. They'll be fun, fast and effective. But when you reach an exercise that's difficult, don't default back to what you know or avoid the learning curve. Be patient and follow this guide with complete trust. Your faith will be rewarded with reshaped abs, bum and thighs – and the confidence of knowing that you finally cracked the weight-loss code.

Once you've completed two or three of the workouts in this book, you can start mixing things up by creating your own. The golden rule is to ensure you work every body part in any given week. So that means you need at least one move from each chapter in Part Two. This will ensure you build a balanced, injury-free body. Working multiple muscle groups also maximises you fat-burning: the more muscle you work the more calories are required both during the workout and afterwards, as your body repairs itself. Furthermore, try to include some workouts with hardly any rest between moves: these will raise your heart-rate and help ramp up your cardio fitness. The bottom line is to make sure you keep challenging yourself. An easy workout is not going to deliver results. And even a tough workout needs to be switched after a maximum of six weeks, to keep your body guessing and therefore changing. Turn to page 222 for a blank chart you can use to make your workouts. But before that, get stuck into one of these.

GLOSSARY OF WORKOUT TERMS

● **Reps**
The number of times you will perform an exercise before taking a break. Sometimes it's time, in which case do as many reps as you can in the time given (or, if it's static, hold the move for that length of time).

● **Sets**
How many times you will repeat a series of reps.

● **Rest periods**
The breaks after each exercise. If no rest and you should move immediately to the next exercise.

● **Superset / Circuit**
This is a group of exercises that are performed with no rest in between. You get a rest once every exercise in the group has been completed.

● **AMAP**
This stands for "as many as possible." Perform as many reps as you can until your form breaks down.

● **Warm-up**
Before each workout, do at least five minutes of warm-up. You can use the bodyweight one in the previous chapter or just jump on the treadmill.

191
Smart moves

Last-Minute Beach Body

45 minutes

The best beach workouts are the ones you can create yourself. This plan will have you ready for bikini season in no time by allowing you to select your favourite exercises. Just follow the template and choose the routine you want to melt pounds and trim inches in just four weeks

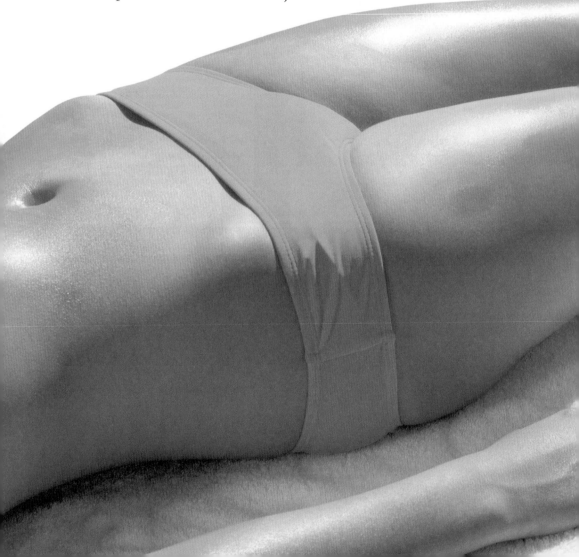

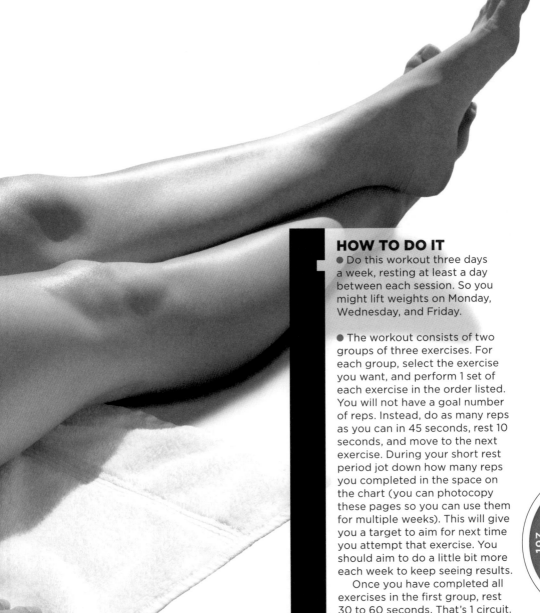

HOW TO DO IT

● Do this workout three days a week, resting at least a day between each session. So you might lift weights on Monday, Wednesday, and Friday.

● The workout consists of two groups of three exercises. For each group, select the exercise you want, and perform 1 set of each exercise in the order listed. You will not have a goal number of reps. Instead, do as many reps as you can in 45 seconds, rest 10 seconds, and move to the next exercise. During your short rest period jot down how many reps you completed in the space on the chart (you can photocopy these pages so you can use them for multiple weeks). This will give you a target to aim for next time you attempt that exercise. You should aim to do a little bit more each week to keep seeing results.

Once you have completed all exercises in the first group, rest 30 to 60 seconds. That's 1 circuit. Perform a total of 6 circuits of Group 1, and then move on to Group 2. Continue this pattern for the second group.

193
Beach body

Beach Body: Group One
(6x45sec sets per move)

		WEEK 1	WEEK 2	WEEK 3	WEEK 4
EXERCISE 1: BACK AND GLUTES					
Deadlift, p141	MON	Exercise: Weight: Reps:	Exercise: Weight: Reps:	Exercise: Weight: Reps:	Exercise: Weight: Reps:
Dumbbell swing, p115	WED	Exercise: Weight: Reps:	Exercise: Weight: Reps:	Exercise: Weight: Reps:	Exercise: Weight: Reps:
Dumbbell clean, p116 **Dumbbell snatch,** p114	FRI	Exercise: Weight: Reps:	Exercise: Weight: Reps:	Exercise: Weight: Reps:	Exercise: Weight: Reps:
EXERCISE 2: UPPER BODY		WEEK 1	WEEK 2	WEEK 3	WEEK 4
Push press, p114	MON	Exercise: Weight: Reps:	Exercise: Weight: Reps:	Exercise: Weight: Reps:	Exercise: Weight: Reps:
Press-up row, p88	WED	Exercise: Weight: Reps:	Exercise: Weight: Reps:	Exercise: Weight: Reps:	Exercise: Weight: Reps:
Chest press, p91 **Overhead press,** p108	FRI	Exercise: Weight: Reps:	Exercise: Weight: Reps:	Exercise: Weight: Reps:	Exercise: Weight: Reps:
EXERCISE 3: LOWER BODY		WEEK 1	WEEK 2	WEEK 3	WEEK 4
Squat, p130	MON	Exercise: Weight: Reps:	Exercise: Weight: Reps:	Exercise: Weight: Reps:	Exercise: Weight: Reps:
Split squat, p129	WED	Exercise: Weight: Reps:	Exercise: Weight: Reps:	Exercise: Weight: Reps:	Exercise: Weight: Reps:
Squat thrust, p113 **Lateral lunge,** p144	FRI	Exercise: Weight: Reps:	Exercise: Weight: Reps:	Exercise: Weight: Reps:	Exercise: Weight: Reps:

Women'sHealth

Beach Body: Group Two (6x45sec sets per move)

EXERCISE 1: LOWER BODY

		WEEK 1	WEEK 2	WEEK 3	WEEK 4
Squat, p130	MON	Exercise: Weight: Reps:	Exercise: Weight: Reps:	Exercise: Weight: Reps:	Exercise: Weight: Reps:
Split squat, p129	WED	Exercise: Weight: Reps:	Exercise: Weight: Reps:	Exercise: Weight: Reps:	Exercise: Weight: Reps:
Squat thrust, p113 **Lateral lunge,** p144	FRI	Exercise: Weight: Reps:	Exercise: Weight: Reps:	Exercise: Weight: Reps:	Exercise: Weight: Reps:

EXERCISE 2: BACK AND GLUTES

		WEEK 1	WEEK 2	WEEK 3	WEEK 4
Deadlift, p141	MON	Exercise: Weight: Reps:	Exercise: Weight: Reps:	Exercise: Weight: Reps:	Exercise: Weight: Reps:
Dumbbell row, p95 **Dumbbell swing,** p115	WED	Exercise: Weight: Reps:	Exercise: Weight: Reps:	Exercise: Weight: Reps:	Exercise: Weight: Reps:
Dumbbell high pull, p116	FRI	Exercise: Weight: Reps:	Exercise: Weight: Reps:	Exercise: Weight: Reps:	Exercise: Weight: Reps:

EXERCISE 3: UPPER BODY

		WEEK 1	WEEK 2	WEEK 3	WEEK 4
Press-up row, p88	MON	Exercise: Weight: Reps:	Exercise: Weight: Reps:	Exercise: Weight: Reps:	Exercise: Weight: Reps:
Incline press, p91 **Overhead press,** p108	WED	Exercise: Weight: Reps:	Exercise: Weight: Reps:	Exercise: Weight: Reps:	Exercise: Weight: Reps:
Push press, p114	FRI	Exercise: Weight: Reps:	Exercise: Weight: Reps:	Exercise: Weight: Reps:	Exercise: Weight: Reps:

Skinny Jeans Workout

30 minutes

Forget fitting into your old jeans. Save up because you're going to need a new wardrobe after this six-week plan. Created by Nick Tumminello, founder of Performance University, this workout burns serious calories. You'll outsmart fat and have the tight, toned look that once seemed impossible

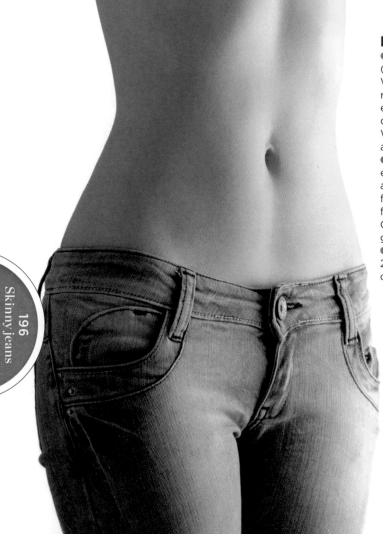

HOW TO DO IT

● Do each weight workout (Workout One, Workout Two, Workout Three) once a week, resting for at least a day after each session. So you might do Workout One on Monday, Workout Two on Wednesday, and Workout Three on Friday.

● Perform each 'superset' pair of exercises back-to-back without any rest. After you complete the final exercise in the pairing, rest for 60 seconds, and repeat. Once you finish all sets in each group, then move on.

● For accelerated fat loss, add 20 minutes of the cardio of your choice at the end of the workout.

Women'sHealth — Skinny Jeans Workout One

SUPERSET A

Exercise		WEEK 1	WEEK 2	WEEK 3	WEEK 4	WEEK 5	WEEK 6
Shoulder Press, p109 — 3 sets, 8-12 reps	Weight						
	Reps						
Swiss Ball Leg Curl, p145 — 3 sets, 15-20 reps	Weight						
	Reps						

SUPERSET B

Exercise		WEEK 1	WEEK 2	WEEK 3	WEEK 4	WEEK 5	WEEK 6
Press-Ups, p83 — 3 sets, AMAP	Reps						
Side Crunches, p148 — 3 sets, 8-12 reps	Reps						

SUPERSET C

Exercise		WEEK 1	WEEK 2	WEEK 3	WEEK 4	WEEK 5	WEEK 6
Incline Press, p91 — 3 sets, 8-12 reps	Weight						
	Reps						
Low Cable Chops, p159 — 3 sets, 12-15 reps	Weight						
	Reps						

SUPERSET D

Exercise		WEEK 1	WEEK 2	WEEK 3	WEEK 4	WEEK 5	WEEK 6
Lateral Shoulder Raise, p105 — 3 sets, 10-12 reps	Weight						
	Reps						
Overhead Tricep Extensions, p101 — 3 sets, 10-12 reps	Weight						
	Reps						

197
Skinny jeans

Skinny Jeans Workout Two

		WEEK 1	WEEK 2	WEEK 3	WEEK 4	WEEK 5	WEEK 6
SUPERSET A							
Barbell Squat, p127 6 sets, 45sec	Weight						
	Reps						
Swiss Ball Crunches, p148 6 sets, 45sec	Weight						
	Reps						
SUPERSET B							
Lunges, p136 6 sets, 45sec	Weight						
	Reps						
Dumbbell Side Bend, p164 6 sets, 45sec	Weight						
	Reps						
SUPERSET C							
Romanian Deadlift, p140 6 sets, 45sec	Weight						
	Reps						
Band Tight Rotation, p158 6 sets, 45sec	Reps						
SUPERSET D							
Barbell Hip Raise, p142 6 sets, 45sec	Weight						
	Reps						
Swiss Ball Leg Curl, p145 6 sets, 45sec	Reps						

Women'sHealth

Skinny Jeans Workout Three

		WEEK 1	WEEK 2	WEEK 3	WEEK 4	WEEK 5	WEEK 6
SUPERSET A							
Barbell Bow, p93 6 sets, 45sec	Weight						
	Reps						
Jackknife, p161 6 sets, 45sec	Reps						
SUPERSET B							
Inverted Row, p93 6 sets, 45sec	Reps						
Decline Side Plank, p151 6 sets, 45sec	Time						
SUPERSET C							
Lat Pulldown, p98 6 sets, 45sec	Weight						
	Reps						
Low Cable Chops, p159 6 sets, 45sec	Weight						
	Reps						
SUPERSET D							
Lateral Raise, p106 6 sets, 45sec	Weight						
	Reps						
Bicep Curl, p101 6 sets, 45sec	Weight						
	Reps						

199
Skinny jeans

Hollywood Workout

60 minutes

Jennifer Garner. Jessica Biel. Reese Witherspoon. What these women have in common? Valerie Waters. Considered the ultimate Hollywood trainer, Val knows how to transform people – including you. This workout is designed to fit around a busy life, getting you lean, sexy and strong as quickly as possible.

HOW TO DO IT

● Perform this workout three times a week with at least a day's rest between (eg Monday, Wendesday and Friday). Each workout consists of three circuits. Perform one set of all of the exercises in Circuit One, resting 30 seconds between each move. Once you have finished all exercises in the circuit, repeat the process. After you complete all sets move to Circuit Two and finally Circuit Three. You'll be red-carpet ready in four weeks!

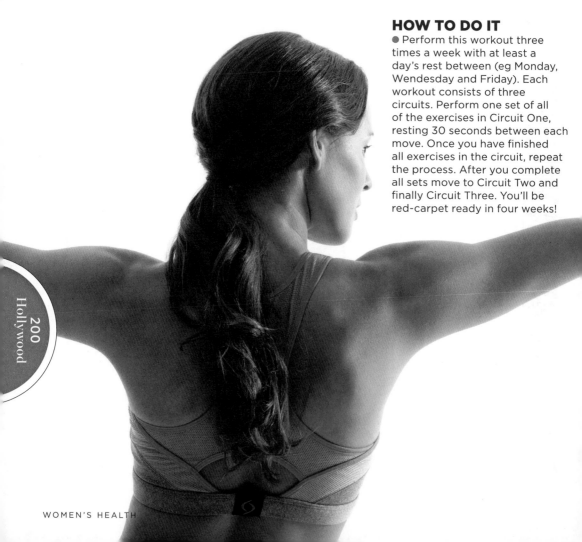

WomensHealth

Hollywood Circuit One

		WEEK 1		WEEK 2		WEEK 3		WEEK 4	
Lateral Band Walk, p144 3 sets, 20 seconds	MON	Reps		Reps		Reps		Reps	
	WED								
	FRI								
Skater Jumps, p134 3 sets, 20 seconds	MON	Reps		Reps		Reps		Reps	
	WED								
	FRI								
Dumbbell Reverse Lunge, p137 3 sets, 20 seconds	MON	Weight	Reps	Weight	Reps	Weight	Reps	Weight	Reps
	WED								
	FRI								
Dumbbell Row, p95 3 sets, 15 reps	MON	Weight	Reps	Weight	Reps	Weight	Reps	Weight	Reps
	WED								
	FRI								
Chest Press, p91 3 sets, 15–20 reps	MON	Weight	Reps	Weight	Reps	Weight	Reps	Weight	Reps
	WED								
	FRI								
Extended Plank, p155 3 sets, 45 sec	MON	Reps		Reps		Reps		Reps	
	WED								
	FRI								

201
Hollywood

Women'sHealth

Hollywood Circuit Two

		WEEK 1		WEEK 2		WEEK 3		WEEK 4	
Lateral Lunge, p144 3 sets, 15 reps	MON	Reps		Reps		Reps		Reps	
	WED								
	FRI								
Dumbbell Push Press, p114 3 sets, 15 reps	MON	Weight	Reps	Weight	Reps	Weight	Reps	Weight	Reps
	WED								
	FRI								
Bicep Curl, p101 3 sets, 15-20 reps	MON	Weight	Reps	Weight	Reps	Weight	Reps	Weight	Reps
	WED								
	FRI								
Dip, p102 3 sets, 12-15 reps	MON	Reps		Reps		Reps		Reps	
	WED								
	FRI								
Mountain Climber, p149 3 sets, 20 reps	MON	Reps		Reps		Reps		Reps	
	WED								
	FRI								

Women'sHealth

Hollywood Circuit Three

		WEEK 1	WEEK 2	WEEK 3	WEEK 4
Single-Leg Hip Raise, p143 2 sets, 15 reps	MON	Reps			
	WED				
	FRI				
Sit-ups, p147 2 sets, 12 reps	MON	Reps			
	WED				
	FRI				
Plank and Reach, p153 2 sets, 20 reps	MON	Reps			
	WED				
	FRI				
Reverse Crunch, p147 2 sets, 15 reps	MON	Reps			
	WED				
	FRI				

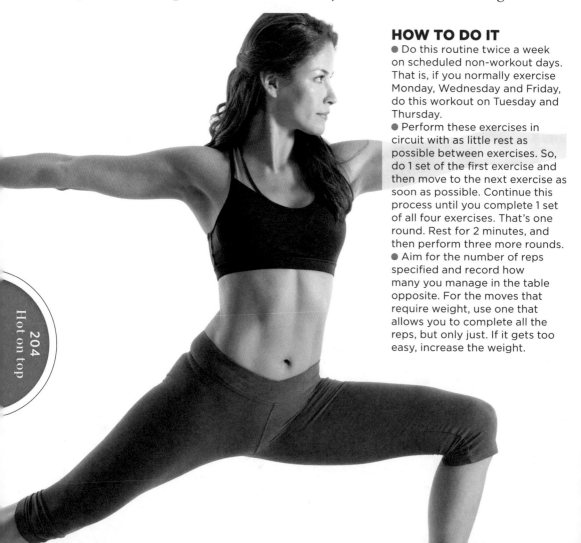

The Look-Hot-on-Top Workout

10–15 minutes

If you want a tight upper body that would make even Rihanna jealous, you need something more than crunches or sit-ups. This workout by Tony Gentilcore, CSCS, might be created by a man, but it's designed to make you a sexier woman. Try out these unique exercises, and then try to tell us that we're wrong.

HOW TO DO IT

● Do this routine twice a week on scheduled non-workout days. That is, if you normally exercise Monday, Wednesday and Friday, do this workout on Tuesday and Thursday.

● Perform these exercises in circuit with as little rest as possible between exercises. So, do 1 set of the first exercise and then move to the next exercise as soon as possible. Continue this process until you complete 1 set of all four exercises. That's one round. Rest for 2 minutes, and then perform three more rounds.

● Aim for the number of reps specified and record how many you manage in the table opposite. For the moves that require weight, use one that allows you to complete all the reps, but only just. If it gets too easy, increase the weight.

Women'sHealth

Look-Hot-on-Top Workout

			WEEK 1	WEEK 2	WEEK 3	WEEK 4
Low Cable Chop, p159 4 sets, 10 reps	TUE	Weight Reps				
	THU	Weight Reps				
Swiss Ball Jacknife, p161 4 sets, 10 reps	TUE	Reps				
	THU	Reps				
Swiss Ball Roll Out, p160 4 sets, 10 reps	TUE	Reps				
	THU	Reps				
One-Arm Farmer's Carry, p123 4 sets, 25 reps	TUE	Weight Reps				
	THU	Weight Reps				

205
Hot on top

Workouts for mums

FROM PREGNANCY TO LOSING THE
BABY WEIGHT, YOU CAN STAY FIT AS
WELL AS BECOMING A MOTHER

Can I work out when I'm pregnant?" It's one of the most common questions from expectant mothers. While your body will go through significant changes, you can still stay fit and help prepare your body for a healthy birth. The secret is a three-step approach that was strategically planned for your changing body and considers all the symptoms you're experiencing. By using this specially designed, workout, you'll gain less fat, suffer fewer aches and pains, and limit your water retention – all while ensuring that you give birth to a healthy baby. And once you have there's another programme to help you shift any baby weight, fast.

THE PREGNANCY WORKOUT: USER'S GUIDE

1 As your belly grows in the second trimester the pressure on your bladder will increase, so it's hard to do "bouncing" exercises like running or jumping.

2 As your abs stretch out, you're going to want to avoid exercises that stretch your abs any further, such as hanging leg raises and leg lowering exercises.

3 Your joints will become progressively looser as your pregnancy continues. So it is wise to avoid single-leg stability work, like single-leg squats or even reverse lunges.

4 It may get harder to squat and deadlift as your hips widen and your belly increases. Assume a wider stance.

5 While your weight goes up, your total strength will seem to go down. If you were used to doing press-ups on your toes, you may be forced into a kneeling position. And chin-ups will obviously be harder as you have more weight to move.

6 Abdominal crunching exercises are not advised as your pregnancy progresses because they can cause Diastasis recti, splitting of your abdominal wall.

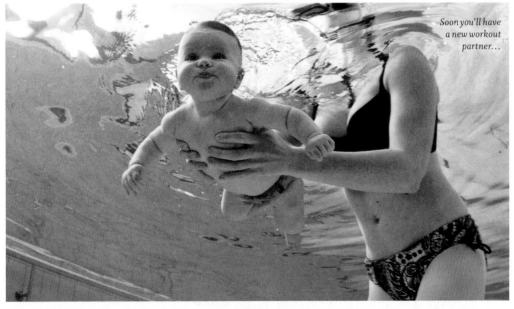

Soon you'll have a new workout partner...

207
For mums

Pre-Baby Phase 1: Weeks 1-15

20-30 minutes

Perform each workout once a week so that you're exercising three days a week. You can switch up the order of workouts or exercises to your preference. Listen to your body during this phase as you're more likely to be excessively tired, nauseated, or wary about exercising in general. Your workouts are going to involve more rest and less intensity until you get your normal energy back.

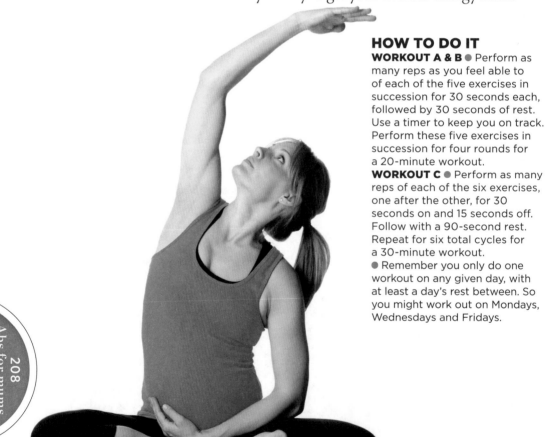

HOW TO DO IT

WORKOUT A & B ● Perform as many reps as you feel able to of each of the five exercises in succession for 30 seconds each, followed by 30 seconds of rest. Use a timer to keep you on track. Perform these five exercises in succession for four rounds for a 20-minute workout.

WORKOUT C ● Perform as many reps of each of the six exercises, one after the other, for 30 seconds on and 15 seconds off. Follow with a 90-second rest. Repeat for six total cycles for a 30-minute workout.

● Remember you only do one workout on any given day, with at least a day's rest between. So you might work out on Mondays, Wednesdays and Fridays.

Pre-Baby Phase One: Workout A

	WK 1/6/11		WK 2/7/12		WK 3/8/13		WK 4/9/14		WK 5/10/15	
	Weight	Reps	Weight	Reps	Weight	Reps	Weight	Reps	Weight	Reps
Goblet Squat, p131 4 sets, 30sec										
Shoulder Press with Twist, p109 4 sets, 30sec										
Hip Raise, p142 4 sets, 30sec										
Inchworm, p122 4 sets, 30sec										
Dumbbell Row, p95 4 sets, 30sec										

209
Abs for mums

Pre-Baby Phase One: Workout B

	WK 1/6/11	WK 2/7/12	WK 3/8/13	WK 4/9/14	WK 5/10/15
	Reps	Reps	Reps	Reps	Reps
Band Squat and Stand, p121 4 sets, 30sec					
Hip Raise, p142 4 sets, 30sec					
Band Squat and Row, p123 4 sets, 30sec					
Band Tight Rotation, p158 4 sets, 30sec					
Forward Punch, p90 4 sets, 30sec					

Pre-Baby Phase One: Workout C

	WK 1/6/11	WK 2/7/12	WK 3/8/13	WK 4/9/14	WK 5/10/15
	Reps	Reps	Reps	Reps	Reps
Squat Jumps, p129 6 sets, 30sec					
Spider-Woman Press-Up, p89 6 sets, 30sec					
Dead Bugs, p164 6 sets, 30sec					
Split Jumps, p135 6 sets, 30sec					
Inverted Row, p93 6 sets, 30sec					
Swiss Ball Rollout, p160 6 sets, 30sec					

211
Abs for mums

Pre-Baby Phase 2 Weeks 16-27

25-30 minutes

By this point, you should really start feeling pregnant. However, now your energy is back and your nausea is gone. So it's time to kick things up a notch and work as hard as your body will let you. As with Phase One you'll do one workout a day, with a day's break between. So you might do Workout A on a Monday, Workout B on a Wednesday and Workout C on a Friday.

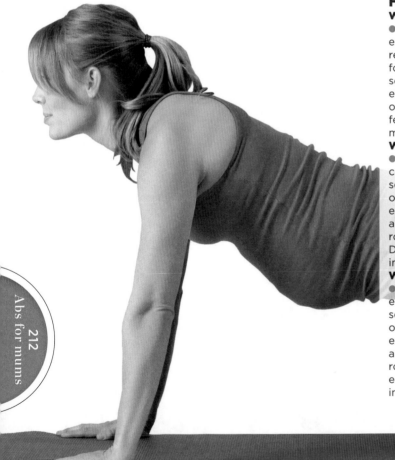

HOW TO DO IT

WORKOUT A
● This workout consists of five exercise pairs. Perform as many reps of an exercise as you can for 30 seconds, then rest for 15 seconds before doing the next exercise in the pair. Do two sets of one pair (or three if you're feeling really energetic) before moving on to the next.

WORKOUT B
● Perform as many reps as you can of each exercise for 60 seconds followed by 60 seconds of rest. Do 1 set of all seven exercises, rest for 60 seconds, and then repeat for three more rounds (four rounds in total). Do each exercise at the highest intensity you are able to.

WORKOUT C
● Perform as many reps of each exercise as you can for 20 seconds followed by 10 seconds of rest. Do 1 set of all seven exercises, rest for 60 seconds, and then repeat for three more rounds (four total rounds). Do each exercise at the highest intensity you are able to.

WomensHealth Pre-Baby Phase Two: Workout A

	WK 16/20/24	WK 17/21/25	WK 18/22/26	WK 19/23/27
PAIR 1				
Stir the pot, p160 2-3 sets, 30sec	Reps	Reps	Reps	Reps
Mountain climber, p156 2-3 sets, 30sec				
PAIR 2				
Side plank (right) p150 2-3 sets, 30sec	Time	Time	Time	Time
Side plank (left) p150 2-3 sets, 30sec				
PAIR 3				
Cable core press (right) p159 2-3 sets, 30sec	Reps	Reps	Reps	Reps
Cable core press (left) p159 2-3 sets, 30sec				
PAIR 4				
One-arm farmer's carry (right) p123 2-3 sets, 30sec	Reps	Reps	Reps	Reps
One-arm farmer's carry (left) p123 2-3 sets, 30sec				
PAIR 5				
Medicine ball side slam (right) p162 2-3 sets, 30sec	Reps	Reps	Reps	Reps
Medicine ball side slam (right) p162 2-3 sets, 30sec				

213
Abs for mums

Pre-Baby Phase Two: Workout B

	WK 16/20/24		WK 17/21/25		WK 18/22/26		WK 19/23/27	
	Weight	Reps	Weight	Reps	Weight	Reps	Weight	Reps
Renegade crawl, p119 4 sets, 60sec								
Squat jump, p129 4 sets, 60sec								
Reverse chops, p158 4 sets, 60sec								
High pull, p116 4 sets, 60sec								
Lateral lunge, p144 4 sets, 60sec								
Dumbbell row, p95 4 sets, 60sec								
Kettlebell windmill, p122 4 sets, 60sec								

Women'sHealth Pre-Baby Phase Two: Workout C

	Reps	WK 16/20/24	WK 17/21/25	WK 18/22/26	WK 19/23/27
Band squat & stand, p121 4 sets, 20sec	Reps				
Resistance band curl, p103 4 sets, 20sec	Reps				
Lateral lunge, p144 4 sets, 20sec	Reps				
Resistance band row, p94 4 sets, 20sec	Reps				
Band overhead press, p103 4 sets, 60sec	Reps				
Band pull-apart p97 4 sets, 60sec	Reps				
Band squat & press, p115 4 sets, 60sec	Reps				

215
Abs for mums

Pre-baby Phase 3: Weeks 28-39

35 minutes

This is it – the last of your glory days. The jumping and explosive moves are going to stop, and you will have a harder time moving your body around. You also will probably find yourself squatting wider and preferring a sumo-style position. But your body is still strong and will amaze you at what it can do. Again, do one workout a day, and three workouts in total each week.

HOW TO DO IT

WORKOUT A ● Perform this workout as straight sets. That is, do 1 set of the first exercise, rest, and do another set of the same one. Continue until you have completed all sets, and then move on to the next exercise. For this workout, you'll perform each exercise for 40 seconds followed by 20 seconds of rest. Complete 5 sets, rest 1 minute, and then move on to the next exercise.

WORKOUT B ● This workout consists of four exercise pairs. Perform as many reps of each exercise as you can for 20 seconds and then rest for 10 seconds. Do all sets in a pair (exercise 1A and 1B, for example) before moving on to the next group (2A and 2B).

WORKOUT C ● Perform as many reps of each exercise as you can for 30 seconds followed by 15 seconds of rest. Do 1 set of all six exercises, rest for 90 seconds, and then repeat for five more rounds (six total rounds). Each exercise is meant to be done at the highest intensity possible.

Women'sHealth

Pre-Baby Phase Three: Workout A

	WK 28/32/36			WK 29/33/37		WK 30/34/39		WK 31/35/39	
	Reps			Reps		Reps		Reps	

Rolling Plank, p154
5 sets, 40sec

Lateral Lunge, p144
5 sets, 40sec

Squat to Overhead Press, p121
5 sets, 40sec
Weight | Reps

Dumbbell Swing, p115
5 sets, 40sec
Weight | Reps

Resistance Band Pulldown, p97
5 sets, 40sec

217
Abs for mums

Pre-Baby Phase Three: Workout B

	WK 28/32/36		WK 29/33/37		WK 30/34/38		WK 31/35/39	
	Reps							
Plank and Reach (right) p153 4 sets, 20sec								
Plank and Reach (left) p153 4 sets, 20sec								
EXERCISE 2A & 2B								
Low Cable Chop (right) p159 4 sets, 20sec	Weight Reps		Weight		Weight		Weight	
Low Cable Chop, (left) p159 4 sets, 20sec	Weight Reps		Weight		Weight		Weight	
EXERCISE 3A & 3B								
Sumo Front Squat, p128 4 sets, 20sec	Weight Reps		Weight		Weight		Weight	
One-Arm Farmer's Carry, p123 4 sets, 20sec	Weight Reps		Weight		Weight		Weight	
EXERCISE 4A & 4B								
Windmill (right) p122 4 sets, 20sec	Weight Reps		Weight		Weight		Weight	
Windmill (left) p122 4 sets, 20sec								

Women'sHealth — *Pre-Baby Phase Three: Workout C*

	WK 28/32/36		WK 29/33/37		WK 30/34/38		WK 31/35/39	
	Weight	Reps	Weight	Reps	Weight	Reps	Weight	Reps
Sumo Deadlift, p140 — 6 sets, 30sec								
Press-Ups, p83 — 6 sets, 30sec								
Plank, p150 — 6 sets, 30sec								
Hip Raise, p142 — 6 sets, 30sec								
Resistance Band Row, p94 — 6 sets, 30sec								
Band Overhead Press, p103 — 6 sets, 30sec								

219
Abs for mums

Lose-the-Baby-Weight Workout

35-40 minutes

After your baby is born, you're thrilled with the new addition to your family but not the changes to your wardrobe. If you want the weight gone fast follow this routine created by Patrick Striet, CSCS, based on the concept of tri-sets. Each tri-set consists of three exercises: one upper body, one lower body and one for your core. Tri-sets will enable you to drop pounds like never before.

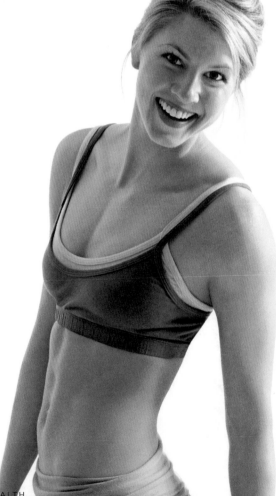

HOW TO DO IT

● Perform this workout 3 days a week on non-consecutive days (Monday, Wednesday, and Friday for example). For each tri-set, perform a set of exercise A, followed by a set of exercise B, and finally a set of exercise C, resting only 45 seconds between exercises. Once you have completed all of the sets in a group, rest 90 seconds and then move to the next tri-set.

Women'sHealth — Lose-The-Baby-Weight Workout

		WEEK 1			WEEK 2			WEEK 3		
		MON	WED	FRI	MON	WED	FRI	MON	WED	FRI
TRI-SET 1										
Overhead press p108 2 sets, 9-12 reps	Weight									
	Reps									
Goblet lunge p137 2 sets, 9-12 reps	Weight									
	Reps									
One-arm carry p123 2 sets, 60 feet	Weight									
	Distance									
TRI-SET 2										
One-arm row p96 2 sets, 9-12 reps	Weight									
	Reps									
Swiss ball leg curl p145 2 sets, 12-15 reps	Reps									
One-leg plank, p154 2 sets, 12-15 reps	Time									
TRI-SET 3										
Incline press-up p88 2 sets, 12-15 reps	Reps									
Goblet squat p131 2 sets, 12-15 reps	Weight									
	Reps									
Cable core press p159 2 sets, 9-12 reps	Weight									
	Reps									
TRI-SET 4										
Resistance band pulldown p97 2 sets, 9-12 reps	Reps									
Romanian deadlift p140 2 sets, 9-12 reps	Weight									
	Reps									
Swiss ball jackknife p161 2 sets, 9-12 reps	Reps									

221
Abs for mums

Women'sHealth

		WEEK 1		WEEK 2		WEEK 3		WEEK 4	
		Weight	Reps	Weight	Reps	Weight	Reps	Weight	Reps
EXERCISE	MON								
	WED								
	FRI								
EXERCISE	MON								
	WED								
	FRI								
EXERCISE	MON								
	WED								
	FRI								
EXERCISE	MON								
	WED								
	FRI								
EXERCISE	MON								
	WED								
	FRI								

BUILD YOUR OWN WORKOUT

EXERCISE		WEEK 1		WEEK 2		WEEK 3		WEEK 4	
		Weight	Reps	Weight	Reps	Weight	Reps	Weight	Reps
	MON								
	WED								
	FRI								
EXERCISE		Weight	Reps	Weight	Reps	Weight	Reps	Weight	Reps
	MON								
	WED								
	FRI								
EXERCISE		Weight	Reps	Weight	Reps	Weight	Reps	Weight	Reps
	MON								
	WED								
	FRI								
EXERCISE		Weight	Reps	Weight	Reps	Weight	Reps	Weight	Reps
	MON								
	WED								
	FRI								
EXERCISE		Weight	Reps	Weight	Reps	Weight	Reps	Weight	Reps
	MON								
	WED								
	FRI								

INDEX

WOMEN'S HEALTH